KETO DESSERTS COOKBOOK

- 2021 -

For a Healthy and Carefree Life.

200+ Quick and Easy Ketogenic Bombs, Cakes, and Sweets to Help You Lose Weight, Stay Healthy, and Boost Your Energy without Guilt

By

Isabelle Lauren

Table of Contents

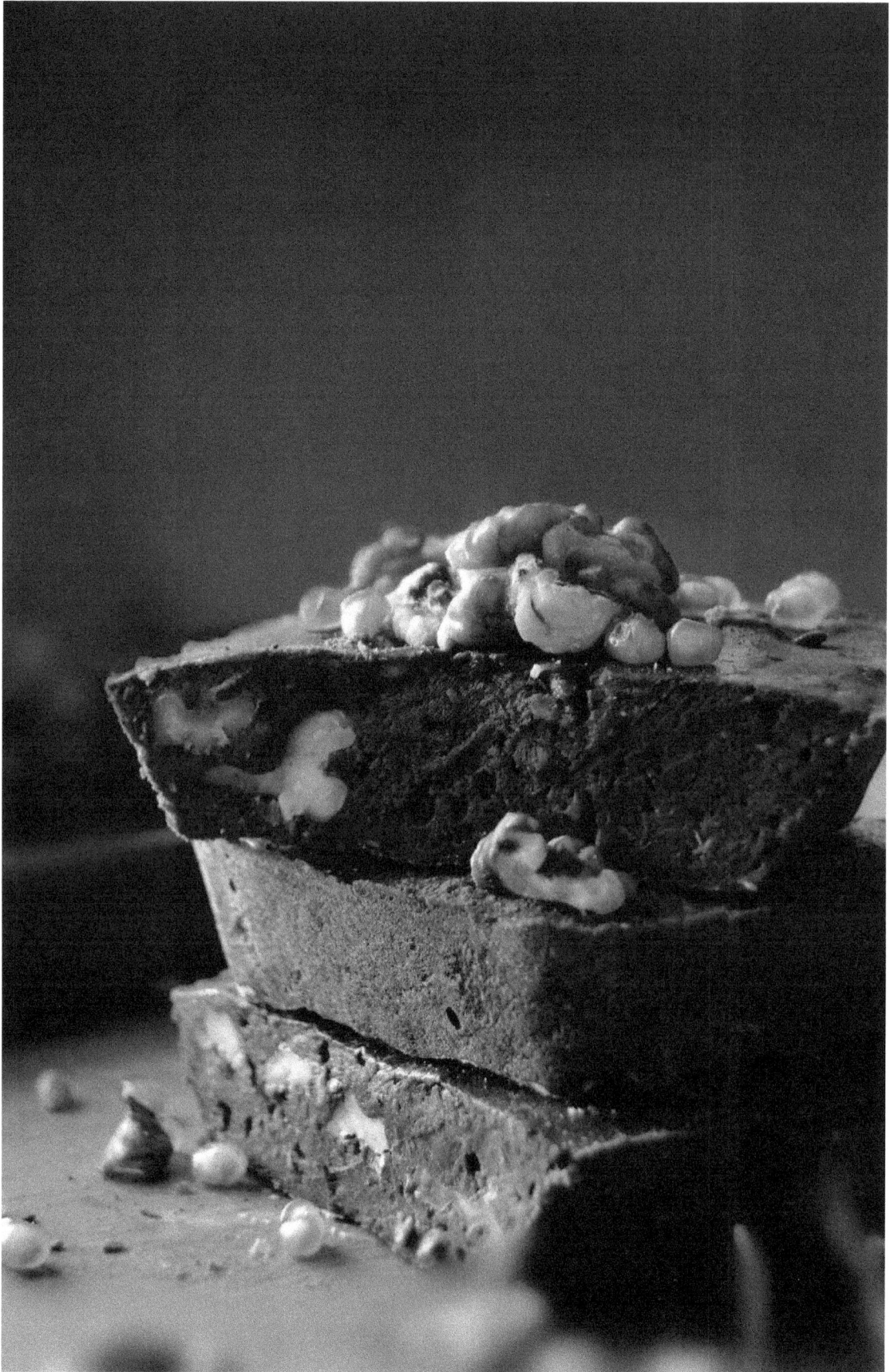

Introduction

Using a metabolic switch in the primary cellular fuel source to which your body and brain are adapted, a ketogenic diet plan improves your health. When your metabolism shifts to fat-based fuels and fat metabolism products called ketones from relying on carbohydrate-based fuels (starch and sugar glucose), positive changes occur at the cellular level, resulting in better overall health.

It is the responsibility of a metabolic process called ketogenesis and a body state called ketosis. Ketosis is simply a normal metabolic pathway in which ketones are used by body and brain cells to produce energy, rather than relying solely on sugar (i.e. carbohydrates). In fact, as an adaptation to periods of food scarcity, humans developed an evolutionary ability to burn ketones.

The ketogenic diet has been used in medicine for over half a century, although it has been more commonly known for several years. The introduction into the ketosis state of patients with neurodegenerative diseases can result in a significant health improvement that applies to epilepsy or Alzheimer's disease. Furthermore, people who want to reduce body weight, but have failed to achieve this objective on a high-fat diet are increasingly using the ketogenic diet. When a major nutritional problem is the excess calories consumed by Europeans, ketosis can be an effective way to eliminate a large proportion of products, which helps many people maintain a certain caloric regime. Besides, metabolic changes occurring during ketosis can promote fat burning and decrease the level of blood insulin,

Is ketosis a remedy for the obesity problem and other diet-related diseases of today? Or maybe its efficacy is only based on the caloric deficit, which is easier to achieve if we eliminate from our diet a large group of products?

Weight loss with fat bombs? Granted, that, at first, sounds funny.

Because we think of cream pie, pizza, doughnuts & Co. immediately with calorie bombs. But we mean "fat bombs" when we say fat bombs: small balls made of a combination of high-fat and low-carb components. Butter, cream, coconut oil, and nuts (and often chocolate-YAY!), for instance.

One may not believe it, but even part of a diet is the little treats. High fat, moderate protein, and low carbohydrates are the basis of the Ketogenic diet or Keto diet for short.

Fat bombs, best of all, are super-fast and easy to prepare. And truly handy on the go as a snack.

You should not overdo it, of course, and eat five at once. But fat bombs are produced from good fats and can effectively help you lose weight. We remain full longer and have no food cravings, thanks to the tiny super balls.

Chapter One. Keto Diet and Dessert Philosophy

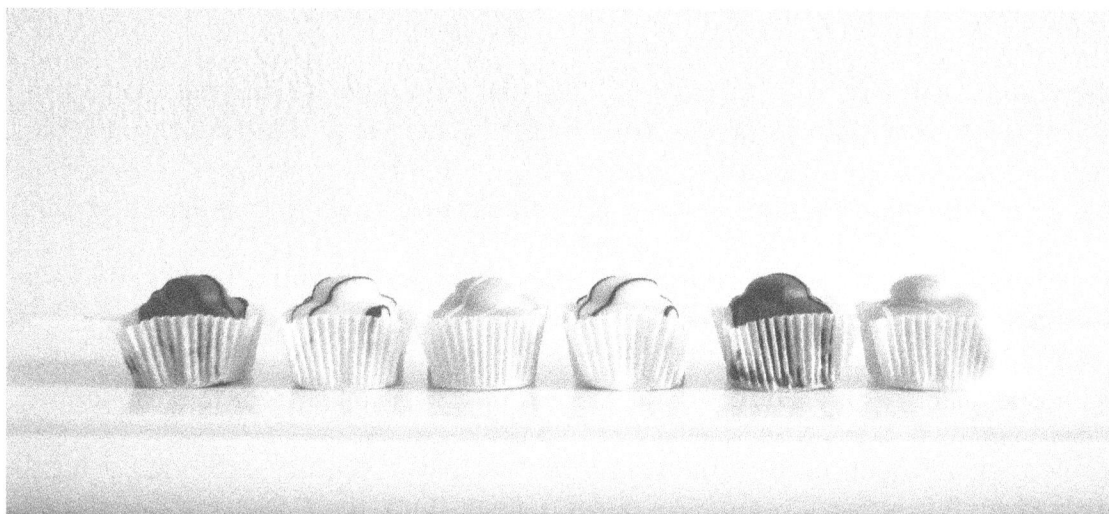

The ketogenic diet is gaining popularity as with "little effort," people can lose large amounts of weight, especially fat. But how healthy is it?

A ketogenic diet gets its name because, through eating, you put the body into ketosis. To understand what ketosis is, you must know that the body mainly feeds on glucose (carbohydrates) and, when you deprive it of its main source of energy, it begins to feed mainly on ketone bodies or ketones, which are produced when fat is oxidized; that is, go into ketosis.

The body is wonderful and developed this process in the case at some point in life, there is a shortage of food. This means that your body is not bad with you by storing fat, but rather it does it so that it has something to eat in times of famine. There is currently an excess of calorie-dense and easily accessible foods, which makes it easier to accumulate body fat and gain weight.

Ketosis can occur with a fast or by eating foods that are low in carbohydrates (less than 20 g of carbohydrates per day). Foods of animal origin usually contain minimal or no carbohydrates, which is why the ketogenic diet is usually based on high consumption of these types of products.

At the moment, everything sounds incredible about following a ketogenic diet, but what are the pros and cons?

PROS	CONS
Once you enter ketosis, fat is used as your main source of energy.	During the first few days, the body obtains glucose through amino acid gluconeogenesis, so, likely, you will also lose muscle mass.
When you enter ketosis, your appetite decreases which also causes you to eat less and lose more weight.	Carbohydrates are available in most foods, making this diet difficult to maintain long-term.
It is an effective method in the short and medium-term.	There is no strong scientific evidence to prove it is a good method for long-term weight loss.
There is no limit to the amounts you can eat of carbohydrate-free foods - more fat and protein. (Although, as we mentioned earlier, a lack of appetite usually helps you eat less)	Normally, the most common foods are those of animal origin, which have toxins, hormones and other substances with harmful effects on health. Besides, by eliminating most fruits and vegetables from the diet, deficiencies of essential nutrients for health have been seen only in these foods.

The table above shows only some of the advantages and disadvantages; however, it is important to delve into some of this type of diet's risks.

The ketogenic diet has sometimes been associated with the following adverse effects:

- Lack of concentration and memory.

- Trouble sleeping.

- Headaches.

- Diarrhea / constipation.

- Tachycardia.

- Muscle pains.

- Dizziness.

- Sudden death.

Besides, a study published in the British Journal of Nutrition in 2013 evaluated the effects of the diet of 247 patients who ate a low-carbohydrate diet. This type of diet was found to alter arterial function, as there was a decrease in blood flow. That means that low-carb diets increase cardiovascular risk. This probably occurs due to nutrient deficiencies, such as selenium, and high consumption of fats and proteins of animal origin, which sometimes increase cholesterol levels in people who follow these diets regardless of weight loss.

Low-carbohydrate diets that focus on the consumption of animal products have also been linked to a higher number of deaths from cardiovascular disease and cancer.

Due to these negative effects of the ketogenic diet, we must be careful when doing this type of diet and always go to a health professional to avoid damaging our body.

The Vegan Ketogenic Diet, is it Better?

Many times, the problem of the ketogenic diet is the excessive consumption of fats and proteins of animal origin such as meat, chicken, fish, sausages, etc. These products often fill us with toxins and hormones that cause imbalances in our body and can trigger chronic diseases.

There is a variation of the ketogenic or low carb diet, where only plant-based foods are consumed. This is quite restrictive, as plant-based foods tend to have a higher carbohydrate concentration, so the main foods consumed to achieve a low-carbohydrate diet are avocados, nuts, seeds, vegetables, and soy (tofu or tempeh), processed meat or sausages, oils, etc.

This type of vegan ketogenic diet was evaluated in 2009 by researchers at a hospital in Toronto, Canada. Even though the sample of patients was small and the study duration was short, the results showed that this type of diet had a reduction in mortality from all causes compared to a low-carbohydrate diet consuming animal product, where it does increase all-cause mortality.

Despite the favorable results of the previous study, it is much better to eat a diet based on plants and natural foods than a vegan diet high in processed products.

So, is it Good to Go on a Ketogenic Diet?

In conclusion, the ketogenic diet has several benefits, especially related to weight loss. Still, it is not because the diet itself is healthy, but because losing weight in overweight or obese people will always bring benefits.

Suppose you are interested in losing weight or improving your health. In that case, it is advisable to change your habits and start following an EAT CLEAN philosophy instead of going on a diet that will probably bring you more problems in the future. Consuming more natural and plant-based foods, as well as significantly reducing the consumption of processed foods, will make you achieve an adequate weight without much effort, will make you feel more energetic, happier and will improve your health in the short and long term.

Is It Good to Eat Desserts on the Keto Diet

The keto diet is a great way to lose weight and sensitize cells to insulin if we are prediabetic or diabetic. Many people join this diet because it gets great results, and because you can do a lot of sweet things that "don't get fat."

But aren't these desserts fattening? Is it a good idea to eat them regularly? In this post, I analyse the pros and cons of eating keto desserts and my personal experience with them.

Before analysing the pros and cons, I would like to make one thing clear, no food does not make you fat. Unfortunately, the internet is full of recipes for keto desserts with titles like fat burning cake or fat-burning ice cream. Please stop this fat burning food stupidity; there is no fat burning food, that's just plain ridiculous. Anything we eat starts the energy-saving mechanism, because it is the way the body works. Fattening or not depends on whether we make use of that stored energy or not. Now, if we are going to see the pros and cons!

Pros

They Are a Much Healthier Option to Conventional Desserts

A keto dessert will always be much healthier than a conventional dessert. Traditional desserts raise and lower glucose and insulin in the blood, which then creates a drop in sugar, leading people to eat continuously.

Keto desserts, on the other hand, being made from low-carb flours do not produce these glucose and insulin highs and lows. Besides, being made of fat and protein, the person is so satiated that it is impossible to eat much. Carbohydrates enter easily because they are easy to digest. Still, protein that costs more to digest does not because it has to be broken down first in the stomach.

They Help Us at the Beginning of the Transition

Depending on what type of diet a person is on, keto desserts can be a good way to transition to a better diet.

If a person comes from a diet loaded with desserts, cakes and candies and tries to leave them overnight, it will be very difficult, and it will be almost impossible for them to stay committed to their new healthy eating plan. This is where keto desserts are a very good thing to include, as they will satisfy that craving without sending your blood sugar or insulin skyrocketing.

You have to understand that the process of losing weight is something that affects people psychologically, it is about breaking a pattern of behaviour and even addictions, this is something really difficult to correct for some people.

If someone has a craving, they will end up eating it anyway, in fact, the more something is prohibited, the more they want, and from here then the eating disorders are born, because the person restricts themselves so much that later they consume it because they cannot take it anymore, and then they feel guilty by eating it and creates an unhealthy relationship with food. So, if a keto dessert can alleviate those intense cravings for something sweet without feeling guilty, be it, but you also have to understand that you can't base a diet on them.

It is Delicious

Losing weight and being healthy are two important things in life, but you also have to enjoy it and indulge in certain pleasures. A keto dessert can be the same or better than a conventional dessert, it will be healthier, and it will make us feel good which is important for our mental well-being.

Cons

They Do Not Provide Too Many Nutrients

In general, desserts are not as nutrient-dense as meats and are usually loaded with fat, which is not good if we are looking to lose weight. As much as fat makes you fat less than carbohydrates, it makes you fat anyway; the body is not stupid; if we eat too much, it will save it yes or yes, because its survival depends on it.

They Perpetuate the Bad Habit of Eating Processed Food

A keto dessert is still a processed food, almond or coconut flour is still a processed food because it doesn't grow on trees. Think that to make this flour, you need a lot of almonds, and in nature, it would not be easy to find that amount, so it is not something that we would naturally eat in those quantities.

They Perpetuate the Bad Relationship with Food

If a person has a bad relationship with food, whether it is a love-hate or addiction relationship, continuing to eat this type of food will continue that bad relationship. It can be useful in the transition period, but the idea is to change your mindset and think about food as a way to give your body the best fuel to be and feel in the best possible way, and there are much better foods to achieve this than keto desserts.

They Don't Help You Lose Weight

Suppose after eating your keto dinner you go and binge on keto cheesecake you are not going to lose weight. In that case, it simply cannot be that way because, as I said before, as much as fat does not activate the same hormones to gain weight as carbohydrates, that does not mean that you do not keep it in the Michelin.

Keto Desserts Basic

One of the foods you miss the most is bread when you start a keto, keto, low carb, or low carb diet, right?

Is any solution there? Do we have any alternative that gives us satisfaction, and a clear conscience leaves us?

Do not worry if you dream of taking a bite of delicious bread because I am going to explain how you can eat bread on a diet and some simple and delicious recipes with very few carbohydrates so that they do not get you out of ketosis.

And not only bread... Sponge cake, cookies, muffins, muffins, pizza, pastries, cakes... Well, you can eat a little of it all, but in moderation.

What is the Best Flour for the Keto Diet?

We are used to eating bread made with wheat flour, and in our diets, we have recently introduced other flours such as maize, rye, spelled, etc.

You have certainly also eaten whole-grain breads, multigrain, etc.

Most bread also has other added ingredients.

The issue is that these flours are very high in carbohydrates and have a very high glycemic index, so they are not ketogenic diet friends.

We will look at their nutritional composition to find out which flours we should not use.

How to Use Keto-Safe Flours in Recipes

I recommend that you start by preparing those that are already published and tested if you want to start preparing recipes.

Keep in mind that you do not have to substitute wheat flour for almond flour to achieve good results, but there are more aspects that you should know little by little.

More liquids or fats are typically needed for these flours: eggs, cream cheese, butter, etc. You are going to get the point from them little by little.

The final product will not taste the same as the bread you eat every day, but you can get very satisfying results, and you will enjoy them a lot because you are going to find yourself a lot better.

Where Do You Get These Flours

With a powerful chopper or a food processor, such as a thermomix, you can make almond, linseed, and sesame flour at home. I did not make coconut flour. It is not common in many nations to find them in supermarkets, although it seems that they are already being introduced little by little.

In organic shops and in some herbalists, where it is simpler to find them.

And if not, web-based. You already know that Amazon is very convenient, that it has great prices, and that it takes you home quickly.

We are going to see the features of each of them now.

All about Keto Sweetener

You may find it difficult to give up sweets, especially in the beginning, which is why here is a quick guide to healthy sweeteners you can use, as long as your net carb limit allows.

Stevia

Stevia is used as a sweetener and as a sugar substitute. Stevia belongs to a group of non-nutritive sweeteners. This means that no calories, vitamins, or any other nutrients are present. The availability of Stevia can differ from country to country.

Be careful around sweeteners, especially powdered stevia products, which can also contain artificial sweeteners. These may be the hidden carbs you are eating, which may be the reason why you can't get into ketosis.

Erititol

There is a glycemic index of 0 and 0.2 calories per gramme for erythritol. It does not influence blood sugar and is suitable for a diet low in carbohydrates.

Lohan / Luo Han or Fruits Of The Monk

It is used in traditional Chinese medicine to cure obesity and diabetes. Monk fruit contains compounds that are 300 times sweeter than sugar but have no calories or carbohydrates, called mogrosides. Such mogrosides are extracted from the fruit and marketed as sweeteners for the monk fruit.

Xylitol

It has dental health benefits and can help prevent osteoporosis.

The glycemic index of Xylitol is 13, and it has 3 calories per gramme. If consumed in moderation, it does not significantly influence blood sugar.

Sugar Alcohols

When you look at the label of most sweeteners that contain sugar alcohols, they claim to be "sugar-free" or "carb-free." These products often contain sorbitol and maltitol.

When you come across "zero-carb" products, always be sceptical. There is no set rule for counting carbohydrate content in chicory inulin or sugar alcohols.

My advice is to pay attention to the carbohydrates consumed, even sugar alcohols, as they can disrupt ketosis and weight loss.

Yacòn Syrup

Yacon syrup has long been known for its anti-diabetic properties; it is also high in antioxidants and potassium, which is an essential micronutrient that is needed in greater amounts when it comes to the symptoms of "keto-flu."

Yacon syrup has other health benefits thanks to its important antioxidant properties, and it can help keep your kidneys and gut healthy.

Inulin-Based Sweeteners

Inulin works as a prebiotic, supplying colonic bacteria with food.

For diabetics and those on a low-carb diet, studies show that inulin has a beneficial effect on blood sugar and is one of the best sugar alternatives.

Tagatosa

Tagatose is a substitute for sugar, a monosaccharide that occurs naturally in dairy products, fruits, and cocoa.

Tagatose only has a small effect on blood sugar and insulin levels; it also inhibits digestive enzymes and the breakdown of carbohydrates in the small intestine.

Among other benefits related to the consumption of tagatose are the increase in HDL cholesterol, the prebiotic effect, and the antioxidant effect.

MANNITOL

Mannitol does not affect blood sugar, but in comparison with erythritol, it has more calories, around 1.5 calories per gramme.

According to recent research, mannitol may be a potential treatment for Parkinson's disease. Regarding the side effects, mannitol is not recommended for individuals with anuria and congestive heart failure.

Lyophilized Berry Powder

Berries are generally recognised to be the most nutritious of all fruits and the lowest in net carbohydrates. They add a lot of flavours if you can find freeze-dried berries and powdered berries, and you will only need to use a very small amount, so you do not need to worry about excess carbs.

Lucuma Powder

Lucuma powder tastes similar to apricots, maple, and mango. It is high in carotene and B vitamins, especially B3, potassium, phosphorus, magnesium, and calcium.

Dark Chocolate

Opt for products with more than 75 percent cocoa when looking for high-quality dark chocolate with the least amount of net carbs. I am not interested in a small amount of added sugar, but I avoid products containing certain sugar alcohols that increase blood sugar levels.

The Keto Tools

1. The Scale

It is one of the most important pastry tools in any kitchen. It must be digital since it will give you greater accuracy when weighing the ingredients. It is also preferable that it has the "tare" function (or "tare" in English), which consists of being able to reset the grammes of our scale when we put the container on top so that we only weigh the ingredient that we are going to add. If you do not have this function, you will have to weigh the bowl and then deduct its weight from the total, using math.

2. Balls

We can find them in countless sizes and types, but we will need two. One with about 25 cm diameter and high walls to avoid splashing, ideal for mixing large amounts of dough or beating with electric stirrers. And another smaller size, about 12 cm, for smaller and deep mixes. In this way, instead of spreading through the bottom of our mould, the dough will accumulate in height and beat it much easier for us.

3. Molds

Molds are another essential pastry tool, and without them, we cannot bake! Round, rectangular, plum cake, cupcakes... There is plenty of them, so, depending on the type of mould you think you will get the most out of. This way, you will start having some "basic" moulds to work comfortably with, and you will be able to add more special ones to your collection. The ideal would be to get a pair of basic round moulds (15 and 25 cm) and a mould with cavities for cupcakes; this will solve most of the recipes you want to make. But above all, my advice is to buy some very good quality moulds and take good care of them, so they will be a lifetime investment.

4. Rods And / Or Electric Blender

We always need manual rods on hand to melt chocolate, melt an ingredient, finish mixing a preparation... They are useful for baking and cooking every day.

If we can have an electric mixer with rods, mixing ingredients will be great without effort. They are very useful to prepare any dough, make a buttercream, or mount cream and whites without leaving your arm in the attempt.

5. Siever or Strainer

In baking, sifting the flour in almost all recipes is essential, so we need a sieve or strainer through which the flour can be passed to eliminate possible lumps and impurities. Ideally, our sieve mesh type has a medium size so that the flour is well aerated, separated, and without lumps, but without a long process.

6. Cake Sleeve and Nozzles

If you want to go further in the world of decorated cupcakes, cakes, and cookies, these will be other essential pastry tools. The pastry sleeves will serve to fill, cover or glaze the creams with which we want to decorate our cakes or cookies.

For your convenience, it is recommended to disposable pastry sleeves, especially indicated when we have creams of different flavors and / or colors. These sleeves are plastic triangles to which we only have to cut the tip, put the nozzle that we want and fill them with cream to decorate without having to worry after cleaning them since they are disposable.

7. Grid

They come in various shapes and sizes and their purpose, fundamentally, is to help our preparations cool down well and correctly. The grid allows air to circulate all around the dough, avoiding moisture concentrations in the base of biscuits and cookies (with its consequent "softening"), or that the paper of the cupcakes absorbs the fat and becomes stained. Stackable racks are very useful, especially for cookies, cupcakes or small pastries, which help you save space in the kitchen.

8. Silicone Spatulas

The spatulas will be very good when it comes to scraping the dough or cream bowls, because by attaching themselves completely to the bowl walls, they make it very easy for us to move the doughs in the same container or even incorporate them into a new one. Or mixing ingredients more homogeneously.

There is them with different hardness levels. For example, the harder ones are better to lower dense doughs (like cookies) from bowl walls, and the softer ones are better to scrape the bowls as they conform better to the container's rounded shape. The latter will also be especially good for smoothing filling creams or the surface of our cakes when we want to give it a more casual finish with "imperfections."

9. Roller

For those people who want to get into the world of cookies or decorating with fondant, the rolling pin will be one of their best friends since it is essential to be able to smooth the dough with a uniform thickness.

To achieve better results, many rollers incorporate levelling rings with different heights. In this way, depending on the thickness we want, we will use one ring or another.

10. Baking Paper

Although it is so low, it is a basic of the basics in baking tools. We will use it to bake cookies, line moulds, and even make homemade capsules for our cupcakes and muffins. Luckily, we can find it in any supermarket.

Chapter Two. Candy and Confections

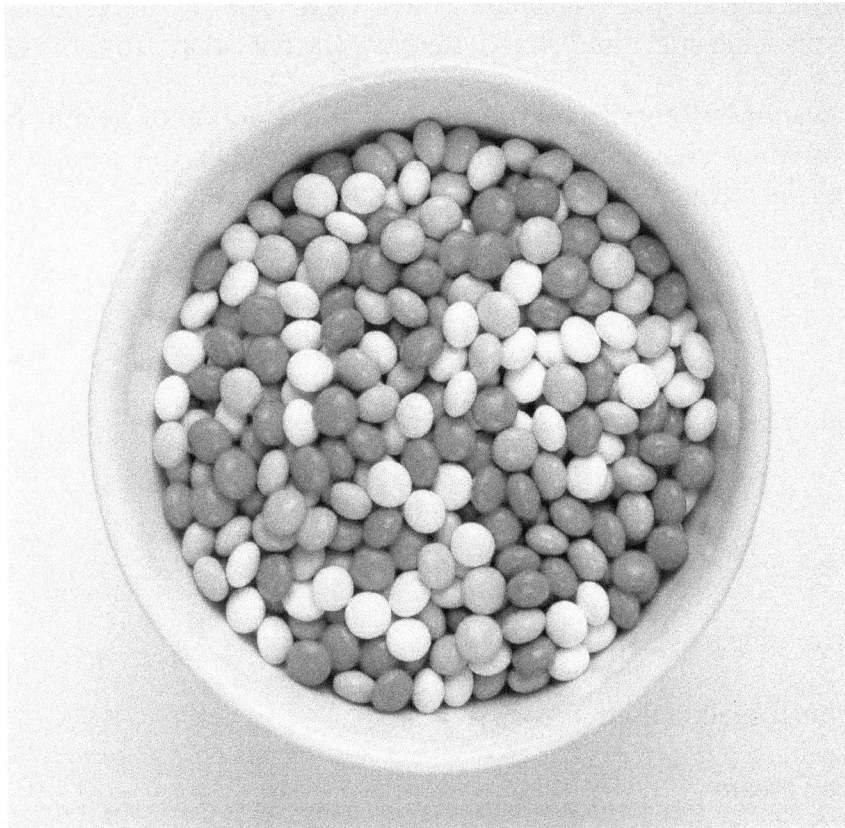

Keto Peanut Butter Cups

Preparation: 20 min ready in 40 min

Ingredients

- ½ vanilla pod

- 60 g cocoa butter

- 50 g cocoa powder (heavily de-oiled)

- 1 tbsp. icing sugar made from erythritol

- 75 g peanut butter

- salt

Preparation steps

1. Halve the vanilla pod lengthways and scrape the vanilla pulp with a knife.

2. Melt the cocoa butter in a saucepan at low heat. Stir in the cocoa powder and vanilla powder. Sift the icing sugar and stir in. Remove the chocolate from the heat.

3. Season the peanut butter with a little salt and add a dollop of peanut butter to each mold. Add the remaining chocolate to the peanut butter. Let the peanut butter cups be set completely in the refrigerator.

Snowballs

Preparation: 40 min ready in 1 h 35 min

Ingredients

- 3 eggs (size m)

- 80 g whole cane sugar

- 100 g wholemeal spelled flour

- 150 g whipped cream

- 1 packet cream stiffener

- 250 g lowfat quark

- 1 tbsp icing sugar made from raw cane sugar

- 1 pinch vanilla powder

- 50 ml apple juice

- 75 g desiccated coconut

Preparation steps

1. A baking sheet with a parchment paper document. Then beat the eggs and whole cane sugar with the hand mixer in 3 minutes until light. The flour all at once admits and folds in. The dough on the plate pass, and in the preheated Backo fen at 180 ° C (circulating air: 160 ° C; gas: Step 2-3) in approx... Bake for 15 minutes until golden. Then take it out and let it cool down for about 30 minutes.

2. For the cream, whip the cream with the cream stiffener until stiff. Cottage cheese, powdered sugar, vanilla powder, and apple juice smooth stirring, then d i.e. Sch l agsahne fold.

3. The cake into small pieces pluck, and the cream gives. Mix everything well. After that, of the mass with a tablespoon 25 portions stab and round shapes. Di e balls in the coconut roll and contact paper cases. Up to Serve cool place.

Chocolate Eggs with Coconut

Preparation: 40 min ready in 2 h 40 min

Ingredients

- 50 g currants

- 3 tbsp. coconut liqueur

- 250 g dark coverture

- 100 ml whipped cream at least 30% fat content

- 2 tbsp. instant coffee

- 80 g soft butter

- 100 g dried coconut flakes

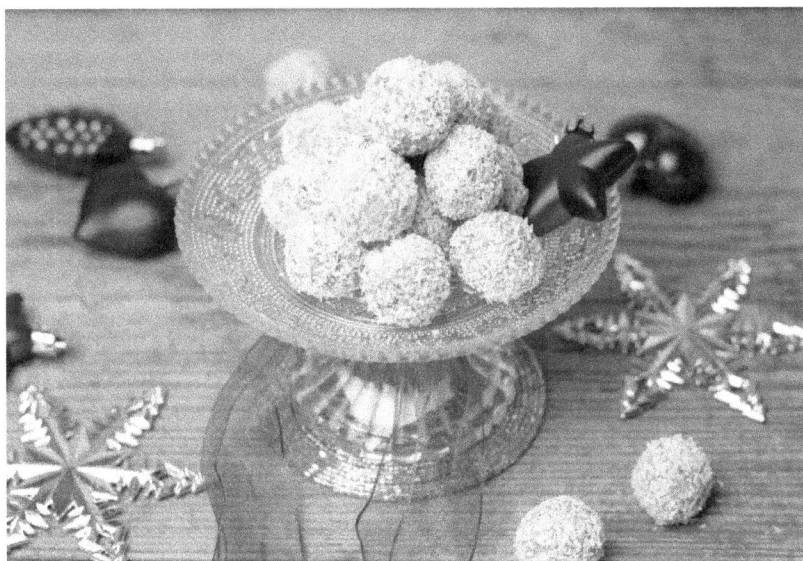

Preparation steps

1. Wash the currants with hot water, drain them well and let them steep in the coconut liqueur in a bowl. Roughly chop the covertures and melt it with the cream and coffee in a saucepan, constantly stirring over low heat, then let cool.

2. Beat the butter until frothy; gradually stir in the cooled chocolate cream. Stir in the currants and about 50 g grated coconut. Cover and chill for approx. 2 hours.

3. Using a teaspoon, cut off small portions of the truffle mixture, shape into oval eggs between the palms of your hands, roll in the remaining desiccated coconut and leave to dry in paper cases. Decorate with bows if you like.

Chocolate and Nut Confectionery

Preparation: 25 min ready in 55 min

Ingredients

- 100 g peanut kernel (shelled)
- 100 g spelled flakes
- 20 pretzel sticks
- 300 g dark chocolate coverture (70% cocoa content)

Preparation steps

1. Roughly chop the peanuts. Slightly crumble the corn flakes. Break the sticks into small pieces (approx. 2 cm).

2. Roughly chop the dark coverture and melt it over a hot, non-boiling water bath.

3. Let the dark coverture cool slightly. Mix in nuts, flakes, and sticks and place small heaps on baking paper with a tablespoon. Let cool and let the confectionery with nuts set.

Chocolate Truffles with a Fine Orange Aroma

Preparation: 1 h ready in 10 h

Ingredients

- 500 g dark coverture
- 75 ml whipped cream
- 1 untreated orange
- 5 drops orange oil pharmacy
- 20 ml orange liqueur
- 60 g soft butter
- cocoa powder for rolling

Preparation steps

1. Finely chop the coverture and place 200 g in a bowl. Bring the cream to the boil, remove from the stove, and pour over the coverture. Wait about 1 minute, and then stir to a smooth mass. Wash the orange with hot water, dry it, and rub the peel finely. Mix with the orange oil and liqueur into the chocolate cream. Cover and let set for about 6 hours.

2. Then add the butter and whisk everything with the whisk of the hand mixer to a light mass. Fill into a piping bag with a small perforated nozzle (approx. 12 mm) and squirt small balls on baking paper. Let it set for about 3 hours.

3. Melt the remaining chocolate over the hot water bath and let it cool down a little. Cover the pralines with the chocolate and immediately roll them in cocoa powder.

Layered Nougat

Preparation: 1 h

Ingredients

- 500 g nougat

- 80 g white chocolate

- 250 g dark nougat paste

- 900 g dark chocolate

Preparation steps

1. Heat (dissolve) the nougat in a water bath to 28 ° C. Chop the white chocolate and melt it in a water bath while stirring until it is 34 ° C. Stir the white chocolate into the nougat. Do the same with the nut nougat and 45 g of dark chocolate.

2. Place two metal strips with a height of at least 2.5 cm parallel to each other on a worktop lined with baking paper. Spread a third of the light nougat in between (approx. 3 mm high). After it has set, spread half of the nut nougat onto the surface of the light nougat and wait until it has cooled down. Repeat this until all the nougat is used up. This results in five layers: three-light and two dark.

3. Let the praline platter harden in about 3 hours. Remove the metal strips. Melt the remaining dark chocolate over a water bath and spread a thin layer on the underside of the plate. Let it become solid. Turn the plate over, coat it with the dark chocolate, let it cool down, and cut into cubes approx. 2.5 x 2.5 cm.

Italian Style Fruit Bread

Preparation: 30 min ready in 1 h

Ingredients

- 300 g peeled nuts (1/3 each of almonds, hazelnuts, walnut kernels)
- 150 g dried fig
- 150 g mixed, candied fruits
- 150 g powdered sugar
- 100 g honey
- baking wafer for laying out the form
- spice mixture 1/4 teaspoon each of cinnamon, clove, coriander, ginger powder, and nutmeg
- 2 tbsp flour
- butter for greasing
- icing sugar for dusting

Preparation steps

1. Preheat the oven to 150 ° C fan oven. Briefly toast the almonds and nuts in a dry pan while stirring. Let cool and roughly chop. Chop the figs and the candied fruits into small cubes, place in a bowl and mix with the nuts with the spices.

2. Place the powdered sugar and honey in a metal bowl on a hot water bath. Stir constantly over low heat until the mixture melts and strings, then let cool a little while stirring. Stir the honey solution into the prepared nut-fruit mixture and mix in 1-2 tablespoons of flour.

3. Brush a flat shape (square or round, depending on the wafers) with butter, line with wafers, pour in the dough, and smooth out. Bake in the preheated oven for about 30 minutes. Let cool down. Dust with powdered sugar to garnish.

Coconut Macaroons with Chocolate

Preparation: 1 h

Ingredients

- 2 proteins
- 100 g fine sugar
- 2 tsp. lemon juice
- 1 pinch salt
- 175 g desiccated coconut
- 200 g dark chocolate coverture

Preparation steps

1. Beat the egg white until stiff; gradually stir in the sugar, lemon juice, and salt. Fold in desiccated coconut with a spatula.

2. Cover the baking sheet with parchment paper. Place small heaps on the tray with two teaspoons. Bake in a preheated oven at 150 degrees (gas: level 1-2, convection: 130 degrees) for about 30 minutes.

3. Let the macaroons cool on a wire rack.

4. Cut the covertures into pieces and place them in a stainless-steel bowl. Melt on a hot water bath, stirring occasionally.

5. Dip the coconut macaroons with the underside approx. 3 mm deep into the covertures, gently wipe the underside on the edge of the bowl, and place the macaroons on a wire rack to dry.

6. Carefully loosen the macaroons with a kitchen knife.

Cheese Cookies

Preparation: 35 min ready in 2 h 50 min

Ingredients

- 100 g cheddar cheese
- 100 g flour
- 1 pinch baking powder
- hot pink paprika powder
- 40 g butter
- 40 g finely chopped pistachios
- 2 tbsp freshly grated parmesan

Preparation steps

1. Grate the cheddar cheese. Mix the flour with baking powder and rose pepper. Add the cheddar cheese and butter in pieces and knead everything until smooth. Finally, work in the pistachios.

2. Shape the dough into a roll (about 5 cm in diameter) and wrap it in aluminum foil. Put in the fridge for 2 hours.

3. Cut the rolling pin into slices about 5-6 mm thick. Place the slices on a parchment-lined baking sheet. Press in lightly with a meat mallet and sprinkle with parmesan. Bake in a preheated oven at 180 degrees (gas: level 2-3, convection: 160 degrees) for 12-15 minutes.

Quince Bread Preserving Sugar

Preparation: 45 min ready in 1 h 50 min

Ingredients

- 700 g quinces
- 300 g apples
- 500 g preserving sugar 2: 1
- sugar to turn

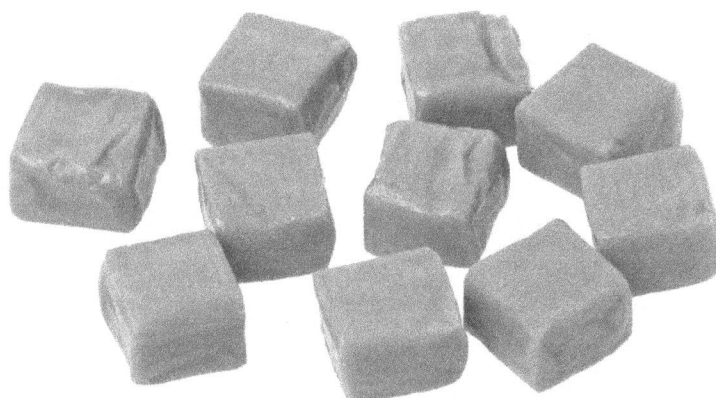

Preparation steps

1. Preheat the oven to 150 ° C top and bottom heat.

2. Quince and apples in quarters and core. Place on a baking sheet lined with baking paper and cook in the preheated oven for 1 hour. Take out and let cool down. Peel the apples and quinces; remove the core, cut into small pieces, then puree. Mix the puree with the preserving sugar, heat, and cook for five minutes. Spread the mixture 1 cm thick on a baking sheet lined with baking paper and let it dry for 2-3 days. Cut into bite-sized squares (approx. 3x3cm) and turn the pieces in granulated sugar. Store hermetically sealed.

Caramel Candies

Preparation: 30 min ready in 6 h 30 min

Ingredients

- 200 ml whipped cream

- 2 tbsp instant mocha

- 200 ml caramel syrup

- 200 g sugar

Preparation steps

1. Bring the cream with the mocha to the boil in a saucepan, remove from the heat, draw and let cool completely.

2. Then pass through a fine sieve and bring to the boil together with the syrup and sugar while stirring and let boil for 10-15.

3. Remove from the heat, place in a tin lined with aluminum foil, spread smoothly, and let cool down. Cut the toffee into cubes and serve.

Heart Chocolates

Preparation: 20 min ready in 2 h 20 min

Ingredients

- 100 g whole milk coverture

- 100 g dark chocolate coverture

- 100 g coconut oil

- 125 ml whipped cream at least 30% fat content

- 50 g nut nougat cream

Preparation steps

1. Cut the two types of coverture and the coconut oil into small pieces. Heat the cream with the coverture, the nut nougat cream, and the coconut oil in a saucepan and melt everything over a medium heat while stirring.

2. Let the mixture cool down a little. Pour the chocolate cream into the molds up to approx. 1 mm below the edge and allow solidifying in the refrigerator.

Caramel Candies (2nd Version)

Preparation: 25 min ready in 40 min

Ingredients

- 200 g sugar

- 150 g honey

- 1 organic orange zest

- 250 ml whipped cream at least 30% fat content

- 50 g butter

Preparation steps

1. Put the sugar, honey, and 5 tablespoons of water in a saucepan and let it simmer for 2-3 minutes. Add the orange peel. Pour the cream into a large saucepan and bring to the boil. Pour in the caramel sugar and cook for about 10 minutes while stirring.

2. As a test, let a few drops of caramel mass drip onto a cool plate or marble board. If the mass becomes firm, it is okay. Stir in the butter. Line a rectangular candy mold (approx. 20x30 cm) with aluminum foil, oil it, pour in the mixture, and allow to cool.

3. Then fall onto a large board and peel off the foil. Divide into candy with an oiled knife. Then let the caramel candies cool down completely.

Toffees with Mocha

Preparation: 30 min ready in 6 h 30 min

Ingredients

- 200 ml whipped cream at least 30% fat content
- 2 tbsp instant mocha
- 200 ml caramel syrup
- 200 g sugar

Preparation steps

1. Bring the cream with the mocha to the boil in a saucepan, remove from the heat, draw and let cool completely.

2. Strain the cream through a fine sieve and bring it to the boil together with the syrup and sugar while stirring and let simmer for about 10-15. Remove from the heat, place in a tin lined with aluminum foil, spread smoothly, and let cool down.

3. Cut the toffee into cubes and serve.

FroYo Bites

Preparation: 5 min ready in 4 h 5 min

Ingredients

- 300 g Greek yogurt
- 1 tbsp. honey (or agave syrup)
- 150 g berries (for example, raspberries or currants)
- 2 tbsp. chopped pistachio
- 2 tbsp. cocoa nibs

Preparation steps

1. Mix the Greek yogurt with the honey and half of the berries. Stir in a tablespoon each of pistachios and cocoa nibs.

2. Now pour the yoghurt mixture into an ice cube container and smooth it out. Then sprinkle with the rest of the berries, pistachios, and cocoa nibs and freeze for around four to five hours.

3. Briefly rinse the back of the ice cube tray under warm water to get the finished FroYo Bites out of the mold more easily and serve immediately!

Frozen Banana Bites

Preparation: 15 minutes ready in 1 h 50 min

Ingredients

- 2 bananas

- 1 ½ tbsp peanut butter

- 70 g dark chocolate coverture (at least 70% cocoa content)

Preparation steps

1. Peel the bananas and cut them into finger-thick slices. Brush half of the banana slices with a little peanut butter and cover with the remaining banana pieces. Put in the freezer for about half an hour.

2. Roughly chop the dark chocolate coverture and slowly melt it over a water bath. Take the frozen banana bites out of the freezer. Dip the banana sandwiches halfway in the melted coverture or drizzle with it, place in the freezer again, and let freeze for about 1 hour. Let the frozen banana bites thaw for about five minutes before serving.

Jelly Bats

Preparation: 15 minutes ready in 3 h 15 min

Ingredients

- 500 ml blueberry juice

- 6 sheets gelatin white

- 1 tube sugar script orange

- 4 silicone or plastic bat molds

Preparation steps

1. Soak the gelatin in plenty of cold water.

2. Heat 100 ml of juice and dissolve the squeezed gelatin in it, mix with the rest of the juice and pour into the cold rinsed molds, put in the refrigerator, and let gel for about 3 hours.

3. Briefly dip the molds in hot water, turn them out onto plates and serve the bats garnished with LM paint.

Walnut Corners

Preparation: 35 min ready in 1 h

Ingredients

- 100 g wholemeal spelled flour

- 140 g butter

- 60 g spelled flour type 1050

- 3 tbsp honey

- 1 vanilla pod

- 1PROTein

- 150 g walnuts

- 100 g coconut blossom sugar

- 50 g whipped cream

Preparation steps

1. For the dough, mix both types of flour, 70 g butter, honey, the pulp of the vanilla pod, and the egg white and knead quickly to form a smooth dough. Shape into a ball and wrap in foil, and place in the refrigerator for 30 minutes.

2. Roll out the dough on a baking sheet lined with baking paper.

3. Roughly chop the walnuts. Heat coconut blossom sugar with 2 tablespoons of water in a small pan and caramelize, stir in walnuts and remaining butter, deglaze with cream and caramelize until golden brown. Spread the walnut mixture on the rolled-out dough and

bake in the preheated oven at 180 ° C (fan oven: 160 ° C; gas: level 2–3) on the lowest rack for approx. 15 minutes, remove, allow to cool, and cut into triangles.

Fudge

Preparation: 2 h 30 min

Ingredients

- 300 g sugar

- 40 g honey

- 5 tbsp water

- 100 g whipped cream

- 50 g dark chocolate

Preparation steps

1. Put sugar, honey, and water in a saucepan and let simmer for 2-3 minutes.

2. Pour the cream into a large saucepan and bring to the boil, dissolve the chocolate in it, then pour in the caramel sugar and cook while stirring until it is brown. This takes about 15-20 minutes.

3. As a test, drip some caramel mixture onto a cool plate to check whether the mixture needs to boil a little or is solid (it should become solid)

4. Line a rectangular shape (approx. 20 x 30 cm) with aluminum foil, oil it, pour in the mixture, and let it cool down. Then fall onto a large board and peel off the foil.

5. Cut out squares with an oiled knife. Let the cream and caramel candies cool down completely. Wrap in corn leaves decoratively as desired.

Sugar-free Fruit Ice Cream

Preparation: 30 min ready in 7 h 30 min

Ingredients

- 60 g large kiwi (1 large kiwi)

- 150 ml clear pear juice

- 1 orange

- 100 g persimmon

- 100 g blackberry

- 100 ml red grape juice

- 100 g strawberries

- 100 ml red currant juice

Preparation steps

1. Peel and puree the kiwi. Mix the kiwi pulp with the pear juice and fill into 4 molds. Halve the orange and squeeze out the juice. Peel the persimmon, cut half into small pieces, and puree the rest with the orange juice. Mix in pieces of persimmon. Pour into another 4 molds and place all ice cream molds in the freezer. Freeze for about 3 hours.

2. For the second layer, wash, clean, and puree the blackberries. Mix the blackberry pulp with the red grape juice. Also wash, clean and puree the strawberries and mix the strawberry pulp with the currant juice.

3. Remove the half-full ice cream molds. Pour the blackberry and grape juice mixture onto the kiwi ice cream. Top up the persimmon ice cream with strawberry and currant puree. Put all ice cream molds back in the freezer and let freeze for another 2 hours. Then stick a wooden handle in each and let freeze for 2 hours.

Chapter Three. Cookies

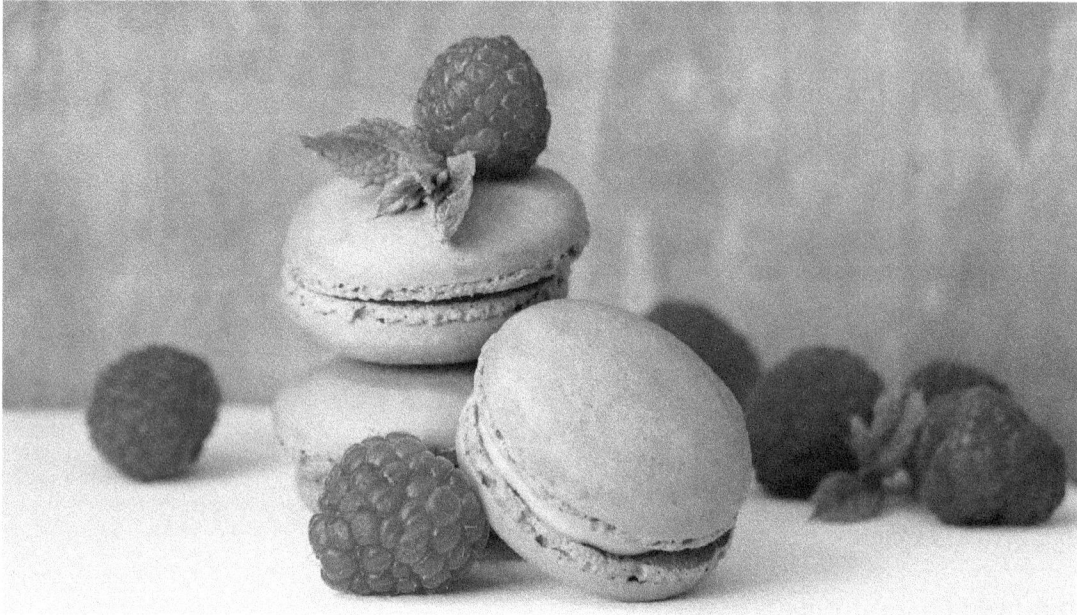

Speculoos Biscuits with Almonds

Preparation: 50 min ready in 2 h

Ingredients

- 125 g soft butter

- 140 g whole cane sugar

- 1 egg (size m)

- 2 tsp ground spekulatius spice (cinnamon, nutmeg, anise, allspice, clove, cardamom, coriander)

- 1 organic lemon (peel)

- 1 pinch deer horn salt

- 3 ½ tbsp milk (1.5% fat)

- salt

- 130 g whole wheat flour

- 120 g wheat flour type 405 + 2 tbsp for processing

- 30 g ground almond

- 80 g sliced almonds

Preparation steps

1. Whisk the butter, sugar, and egg with a hand mixer. Add the speculoos seasoning and lemon zest.

2. Dissolve deer horn salt in 1 tbsp milk and stir in. Add 1 pinch of salt, sifted flour, and ground almonds and knead into a smooth dough. Cover and cool the dough for at least 1 hour.

3. Then knead the dough again, roll it out 3 mm thin on a floured work surface, and cut out rectangles (approx. 4 x 5 cm) with a sharp knife.

4. Place the speculoos on baking sheets lined with baking paper, brush with a little milk and sprinkle with sliced almonds. Bake in a preheated oven at 180 ° C (convection 160 ° C, gas: level 2–3) for 8–10 minutes until crispy. Let cool down completely.

Jam and Coconut Cookies

Preparation: 40 min ready in 1 h

Ingredients

- 2 protein

- 1 pinch salt

- 50 g raw cane sugar

- ½ lemon

- 100 g marzipan paste

- 125 g coconut flakes

- 2 tbsp whole wheat flour

- 125 g raspberry jam

Preparation steps

1. Beat egg whites until stiff. Gradually add salt and raw cane sugar and keep stirring until the snow is very stiff. Squeeze the lemon and melt the juice with the marzipan mixture in a small saucepan, let it cool down a little, and stir into the egg whites with coconut flakes. The result should be soft but malleable dough, stir in a little flour if necessary.

2. Cut off small heaps with two moist teaspoons and place them on a baking tray lined with baking paper, a little apart. Make a small indentation in the middle (e.g. with a wooden spoon handle) and add some jam. Bake in a preheated oven at 160 ° C (convection 140 ° C; gas: level 2) for about 20 minutes until golden brown. Remove from the tray and let cool down.

Raspberry Rascals

Preparation: 30 min ready in 1 h 30 min

Ingredients

- 1 organic lemon

- 250 g spelled flour type 1050

- 50 g ground almond

- 50 g

- honey

- 1 pinch salt

- 1 egg

- 150 g butter (cold)

- 150 g raspberry fruit spread

- icing sugar made from erythritol for dusting

Preparation steps

1. Rinse the lemon with hot water, pat dry, and rub the peel finely. Knead 1/2 teaspoon of the lemon zest, the flour, the almonds, the honey, the salt, the egg, and the butter into a smooth pastry. Wrap it in a cling film and put it in the fridge for about 30 minutes.

2. Roll out the shortened pastry to about 4 mm thick. Cut the cookies with a round cutter (about 4 cm in diameter). Poke half of the cookies in the window with a small star cutter.

3. Put the cookies on a baking sheet lined with baking paper. Bake in a preheated oven at 180 ° C (convection at 160 ° C; gas at 2–3 ° C) for 8–10 minutes.

4. Dust the cookie hole with the powdered sugar of erythritol. Stir the fruit until it is smooth and spread over warm, hollow-free cookies and put together with the other half. Press it lightly and let it cool down. Rascals can be kept dry for two weeks.

Cinnamon Stars Soft

Preparation: 1 h 30 min

Ingredients

- 500 g ground almond kernels

- 5 protein

- 450 g icing sugar made from birch sugar

- 2 tspcinnamon

- 1 organic lemon

Preparation steps

1. Beat the egg whites until stiff and stir in the powdered sugar.

2. Set aside 1 cup of whipped cream for the glass. Rinse the lemon with hot water, pat dry, and fry the peel. Add the almonds, cinnamon, and lemon zest to the whipped cream, knead quickly and cover the dough in the refrigerator for about 1 hour.

3. Roll out the dough about 4 mm thick on the working surface, cut out the stars of different sizes and cover them evenly with the glaze. Place on a baking tray that is covered with baking paper.

4. Bake the cinnamon stars in a preheated oven at 160 ° C (convection: 140 ° C; gas: level 1-2) for about 8 minutes, the stars should remain soft inside, and the surface should remain white.

Oatmeal Cookies

Preparation: 40 min ready in 1 h

Ingredients

- 100 g butter

- 200 g tender oatmeal

- 100 g ground almond kernels

- 50 g wholemeal spelled flour

- 25 g soy flour

- ½ vanilla pod

- 1 pinch salt

- 6 tbsp. honey

- 2 tbsp. milk (1.5% fat)

Preparation steps

1. In a cup, melt the butter, remove it, and let cool a little. In a bowl, mix the oatmeal, the bottomed almonds, flour spelled, soy and salt. Cut off the pulp and add the vanilla pod longitudinally to the dry ingredients.

2. Mix with the butter the sweet and milk. Into the dry ingredients, add the butter mixture, and mix well. If necessary, add a bit more milk. Remove the dough 30 minutes in the fridge.

3. Place little heaps on a breadboard lined with baking paper with a teaspoon, leaving sufficient room for the cookies to break up. In a prehot oven, bake for 5-6 minutes at 220 ° C (fan oven: 200 ° C; gas: 3-4 level).

Cinnamon Cookies

Preparation: 15 minutes ready in 1 h

Ingredients

- 1 short crust pastry (cookie dough according to the basic recipe)

- 20 g liquid butter (2 tbsp.)

- 2 tsp. cinnamon powder

- 15 g raw cane sugar (1 tbsp.)

- 1 egg yolk

Preparation steps

1. First, prepare the dough according to the basic recipe. You can find the link to the "Cookie Dough" recipe under product recommendation or using our search function.

2. Roll out the short crust pastry into a rectangle (about 25 x 40 cm) and brush with the liquid butter. Mix the cinnamon and raw cane sugar and sprinkle with them.

3. Roll up the short crust pastry from the narrow side and refrigerate for another 30 minutes.

4. Cut the short crust roll into 0.5–1 cm thick slices and place on a baking sheet lined with baking paper. Whisk the egg yolk with 1-2 tablespoon of water and brush the cinnamon cookies with it.

5. Bake in a preheated oven at 200 ° C (convection 160 ° C; gas: level 2–3) for 10–12 minutes until golden brown. Take out the cinnamon cookies and let them cool down.

Oat Cookies with Almonds and Walnuts

Preparation: 15 minutes ready in 30 min

Ingredients

- 100 g butter

- 125 g honey

- 1 pinch salt

- 2 eggs

- 200 g wheat flour type 1050

- 1 tsp baking powder

- 100 g tender oatmeal

- 50 g almond flakes

- 50 g chopped walnuts

- 3 tbsp milk (3.5 fat)

Preparation steps

1. Beat the butter with honey and salt until frothy. Gradually stir in the eggs.

2. Mix flour with baking powder and oatmeal and stir in.

3. Add the almonds and walnuts and work everything with a little milk to form a malleable dough.

4. Cut off small heaps from the mixture and place them on a baking sheet lined with baking paper about 4 cm apart.

5. Bake in a preheated oven at 190 ° C (fan oven 160 ° C; gas: level 2-3) until golden brown for about 15 minutes. Take out and let cool on a wire rack.

Chocolate Macaroons

Preparation: 30 min ready in 55 min

Ingredients

- 4 protein

- 2 tsp lemon juice

- 250 g very fine sugar

- 125 g ground almond kernels

- 30 g cocoa powder

For the filling

- 100 g dark coverture

- 2 tbspwhipped cream at least 30% fat content

- 30 g butter

Preparation steps

1. Preheat the oven to 150 ° C fan oven. Beat the egg whites with the lemon juice until very stiff. Gradually pour in the sugar, continue beating until you have a firm, shiny mass.

Carefully fold in the almonds and cocoa. Pour the mixture into a piping bag with a large, round nozzle.

2. Squirt small hemispheres about 2 cm in diameter onto a baking sheet lined with baking paper. Bake the macaroons in the preheated oven for about 25 minutes, leaving the oven door ajar.

3. For the cream filling, chop the coverture into small pieces and carefully melt in a water bath. Mix in the cream and butter in small pieces with the whisk. Let the mixture cool down a little. Brush half of the macaroons with the filling and combine with the remaining macaroons.

Cinnamon Pecan Cookies

Preparation: 45 min ready in 1 h 45 min

Ingredients

- 200 g flour and some flour for the work surface

- 100 g sugar

- 1 pinch salt

- 100 g ground pecans

- 1 tsp cinnamon

- 20 g cocoa powder (1 heaped tablespoon)

- 1 egg

- 200 g yogurt butter

- 55 pecans (half)

- 20 g powdered sugar (2 tbsp.)

Preparation steps

1. Mix the flour with sugar, a pinch of salt, ground pecans, cinnamon, and cocoa powder, pile on a work surface, make a well in the middle and beat in the egg.

2. Spread the yogurt butter in flakes around the cavity. Chop all ingredients with a knife until crumbly. Knead quickly with your hands to form a smooth dough, shape into a ball and wrap in cling film and cool for 30 minutes.

3. Knead the dough again on a floured work surface and divide into 2 portions. Roll out the dough portions into long strands of 2 cm Ø and cut into 1 cm thick slices. Shape these into balls, flatten them slightly, and place them on baking sheets lined with baking paper.

4. Cover the dough balls with 1 pecan half and bake one after the other in a preheated oven at 180 ° C (convection 160 ° C; gas: level 2–3) for 10–12 minutes. Remove the cookies and let them cool down. If you like, you can dust the cookies with powdered sugar.

Jam Cookies with Currant Jelly

Preparation: 30 min ready in 2 h 30 min

Ingredients

- 420 g spelled flour type 1050

- 150 g raw cane sugar

- ½ tsp vanilla

- 1 pinch salt

- 125 g ground hazelnuts

- ½ organic lemon

- 250 g butter

- 2 eggs (size s)

- 200 g currant jelly

- 20 g icing sugar made from raw cane sugar (2 tbsp)

Preparation steps

1. Mix the flour with raw cane sugar, vanilla, a pinch of salt, and hazelnuts in a bowl. Wash the lemon half with hot water, pat dry, rub off the peel and add.

2. Pile the flour mixture on the work surface. Add butter in small pieces, chop in. Add the eggs and quickly knead everything into a smooth dough. Wrap the dough in cling film and let it rest in the refrigerator for at least 30 minutes.

3. Roll out the dough in portions to a thickness of approx. 3 mm, cut out 50 circles and rings and place on baking sheets lined with baking paper. Bake the biscuits one after the other in

a preheated oven at 190 ° C (convection 170 ° C; gas: level 2–3) for 8–10 minutes until they are light yellow and allow to cool on a wire rack.

4. In the meantime, heat the currant jelly in a saucepan. Brush 1 circle with jam on each side and place 1 ring on top. Cool the cookies and let them dry for 1–2 hours. Then dust with powdered sugar.

Chocolate Crinkle Cookies

Preparation: 20 min Ready in 40 min

Ingredients

- 1 shortcrust pastry (cookie dough according to the basic recipe)

- 30 g cocoa powder (4 tbsp)

- 2 tsp gingerbread spice

- 1 tsp baking powder

- 30 g cocoa nibs (2 tbsp)

- 20 g whipped cream (2 tbsp)

- 2 tbsp icing sugar made from raw cane sugar

Preparation steps

1. First, prepare the dough according to the basic recipe. You can find the link to the "Cookie Dough" recipe under product recommendation or using our search function.

2. Mix the cocoa, gingerbread spice, and baking powder. Knead into the short crust pastry together with the cocoa nibs and whipped cream.

3. Shape the short crust pastry into walnut-sized balls, press them flat, roll one side in powdered sugar. Set aside the remaining powdered sugar. Place the chocolate cookies on a baking sheet lined with baking paper.

4. Bake the chocolate biscuits in a preheated oven at 180 ° C (convection 160 ° C; gas: level 2–3) for 15 minutes. Take out and let cool.

5. Dust the chocolate cookies with the rest of the icing sugar before serving.

Chocolate Biscuits

Preparation: 30 min Ready in 1 h 45 min

Ingredients

- 200 g butter

- 2 eggs

- 100 g coconut blossom sugar

- 220 g wholemeal spelt flour

- 1 tsp baking powder

- 2 tbsp cocoa powder

- 50 g ground hazelnuts

- 100 g chopped dark chocolate

Preparation steps

1. Put the butter in a saucepan, melt it and let it cool down again. Beat the eggs with the coconut blossom sugar until frothy. Sieve the flour with the baking powder and cocoa powder over it. Mix in the butter, the ground hazelnuts, and the chocolate. Cover and chill the dough for about 1 hour.

2. Cut off small portions from the dough with a teaspoon and place them on a baking sheet lined with baking paper at a distance of a good 1 cm. Press a little flat and bake in a preheated oven at 200 ° C (fan oven: 180 ° C; gas: level 3) for 10–15 minutes. Carefully remove from the baking sheet and let cool down.

Chocolate Macaroons (2nd Version)

Preparation: 45 min ready in 57 min

Ingredients

- 175 g butter

- 120 g icing sugar made from raw cane sugar

- 1 pinch salt

- 3 eggs

- 175 g spelled flour type 1050

- 125 g ground almond kernels

- 40 g cocoa powder

- 70 g dark chocolate

- 80 g dates

- 100 ml whipped cream

Preparation steps

1. Beat the butter, salt, and sugar until creamy. Beat the butter. Remove the eggs from the flour, almonds, and coconut powder and fold them one by one. Pour the dough into a pipe bag, approximately with a smooth, medium-sized punched nozzle. Three centimeters of a baker on a sheet of bakery. Bake in a preheated oven for 10–12 minutes, remove from the tray carefully, and allow to cool, at 2000C (fan oven: 1800 C; gas level 3).

2. Chop the chocolate roughly to be filled. Stein and purify the dates if necessary. Bring the cream to a boil, remove the chocolate from the heat and let cool until it is spreadable and fold into a mixture of dates. Brush with a little chocolate cream half of the macaroons on the underside, put the remaining macaroons on top, and slightly press.

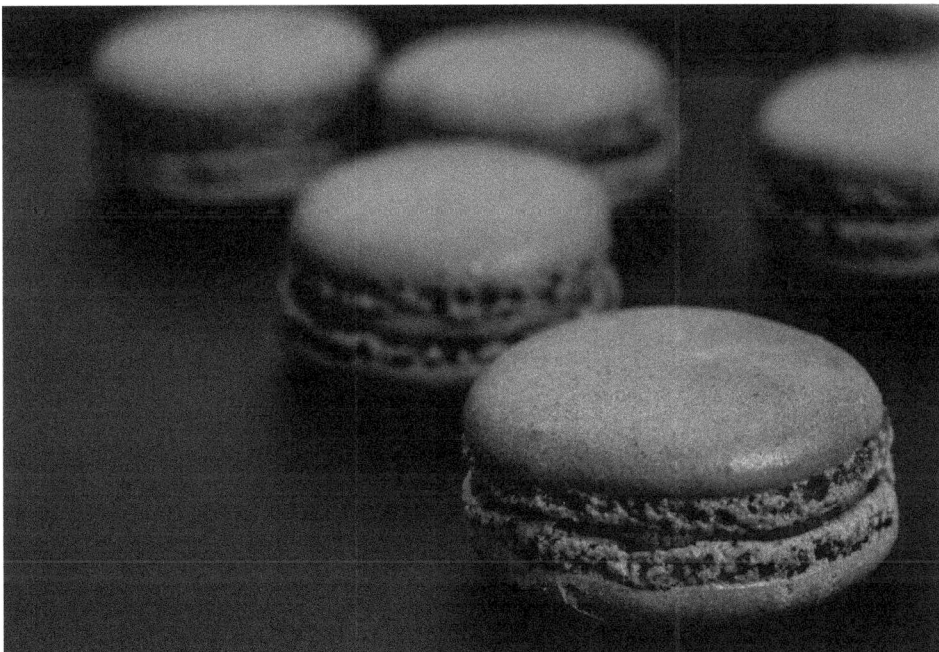

Cinnamon Jam Hearts

Preparation: 45 min

Ingredients

- ½ organic lemons
- 220 g spelled flour type 1050
- 50 g ground hazelnuts
- 60 g cocoa powder
- 120 g whole cane sugar
- ½ tsp gingerbread spice
- 1 tsp baking powder
- 1 pinch salt
- 80 g cold butter
- 1 egg
- ½ tsp vanilla powder
- 1 tsp cinnamon powder
- 100 g strawberry jam

Preparation steps

1. Wash half a lemon with hot water, pat dry; finely grate 1 teaspoon zest (use the rest of the lemon for other purposes). Mix 200 g flour with nuts, cocoa, 80 g whole cane sugar, lemon peel, gingerbread spice, baking powder and a pinch of salt. Add butter and egg, work into a smooth dough; if it is too dry, and knead in water. Shape into a ball and wrap in the fridge for 1 hour.

2. Halve the dough and roll it out 3 mm thick on the floured work surface. Cut out hearts. Place them next to each other on baking sheets lined with baking paper and bake in a preheated oven at 180 ° C (convection 160 ° C; gas: level 2–3) for 10–12 minutes.

3. In the meantime, mix the remaining whole cane sugar with the vanilla powder and cinnamon. Heat the jam and strain it through a sieve.

4. Remove hearts from the tin as hot as possible; Spread half of the jam, place the remaining hearts on top, squeeze gently. Roll in the sugar mixture and allow cooling completely on the wire rack.

Black and White Cookies

Preparation: 45 min

Ingredients

- 1 vanilla pod

- 200 g wholemeal spelled flour

- 100 g spelled flour (type 630)

- 75 g honey

- 175 g butter

- 2 egg yolks

- 2 tbsp cocoa powder

- 2 tbsp whipped cream

Preparation steps

1. The first slit opens the vanilla pod lengthways and scrape out the pulp. Vanilla pulp, both flours, honey, butter, and egg yolks quickly into a smooth shortcrust pastry.

2. Halve the amount of dough and knead under half of the cocoa and cream. Wrap both doughs in cling film and refrigerate for 2 hours.

3. Roll out both doughs about 1.5 cm thick on a floured work surface. Cut into approx. 1.5 cm wide strips and place two white and black strands of dough on top of each other in different colours. Press down well and shape into a square shape. If necessary, brush the edges with a little water so that they stick together better. Cut the ends evenly and wrap in cling film, and put in the fridge for another 30 minutes.

4. Cut 2–3 mm thin slices from the dough, flatten it a little, place on a baking sheet lined with baking paper. Bake in a preheated oven at 180 ° C (convection 160 ° C; gas: level 2–3) for 10–12 minutes until golden brown. Carefully remove from the baking sheet and let cool down.

Hazelnut Cookies

Preparation: 35 min ready in 45 min

Ingredients

- 200 g soft butter

- 150 g whole cane sugar

- 3 eggs

- 280 g wholemeal spelled flour

- 170 g ground hazelnuts

- 2 tsp baking powder

- 3 tbsp cocoa powder

- ½ tsp cinnamon

- 120 ml milk

- 2 tbsp icing sugar made from raw cane sugar

- 1 tsp lemon juice

- 50 g chopped hazelnuts

Preparation steps

1. Beat the butter with a hand mixer until it is frothy. Gradually stir in the sugar. Stir in the eggs one by one and stir for 2 minutes until frothy. Mix the flour with the ground hazelnuts, baking powder, cocoa powder, and cinnamon and stir into the egg mixture alternately with the milk. The dough should fall tough from the spoon.

2. Mix the powdered sugar with the lemon juice and add enough water to make a thin glaze. With a tablespoon, place small heaps on a baking sheet lined with baking paper and spread thinly with the icing. Sprinkle with a few chopped hazelnuts and bake in a preheated oven at 180 ° C (fan oven: 160 ° C; gas: level 2–3) for 10–12 minutes. Remove and let cool on a rack.

Vanilla Crescents

Preparation: 30 min Ready in 2 h 6 min

Ingredients

- 2 vanilla pods

- 280 g wheat flour type 1050

- 100 g ground almond kernels

- 150 g raw cane sugar

- 240 g cold butter

Preparation steps

1. Scrape the pulp and halve the vanilla pods. Knead 260 g of the flour on the surface of the work to form a smooth dough. Knead 50 g of crude cane sugar, flaky butter, and vanilla pulp.

2. Divide the dough on a blurred working surface into 4 portions, form in rolls (2-3 cm in diameter). Wrap and cool for at minimum 1 hour in clinging film. Baked paper cover baking trays. Cover. Thread the rolls around 1 cm thick in 15 pieces. Put them on the tray and shape into croissants. In a preheated stove, cook for about 12 minutes at 180 degrees C, (convection 160 degrees C; gas 2–3). Remove the paper from the tray and turn to still warm the remaining raw cane sugar. Let it refresh.

Cinnamon Cookies with Cream Cheese

Preparation: 20 min

Ready in 3 h 35 min

Ingredients

- 60 g butter (room warm)

- 50 g cream cheese (20% fat in dry matter)

- 1 vanilla pod

- 80 g coconut blossom sugar

- 1 egg yolk

- 130 g wholemeal spelled flour (type 1050)

- 50 g spelled flour (type 630)

- 1 pinch baking powder

- 2 tbsp liquid butter

- 2 tsp cinnamon powder

Preparation steps

1. Whisk the cream cheese together with the butter. Slit the vanilla pod lengthways and scrape out the pulp. Add the vanilla pulp, 50 grams of coconut blossom sugar, and egg yolk. Mix both flours and baking powder and stir in as well. Knead everything into a smooth shortcrust pastry.

2. Roll out the dough between two layers of cling film into a rectangle (approx. 20 x 30 cm). Remove the top foil and brush the dough with the liquid butter. Mix the rest of the coconut blossom sugar with the cinnamon and sprinkle on the dough as well.

3. Use the foil to roll up the rolling pin on the narrow side. Wrap tightly in foil and refrigerate for 3 hours.

4. Line a baking sheet with parchment paper. Remove the foil from the roll and cut into slices about 0.5 cm thick. Place the cookies on the tray. Bake in the preheated oven at 180 ° C (convection 160 ° C; gas: level 2–3) and on the middle rack for about 12 minutes. Take out and let cool.

Chocolate Snowballs

Preparation: 40 min Ready in 2 h 48 min

Ingredients

- 100 g dark chocolate (70% cocoa content)

- 1 vanilla pod

- 150 g wholemeal spelled flour

- 3 tbsp cocoa powder

- 1 tsp baking powder

- 1 pinch salt

- 50 g butter (room warm)

- 60 g honey

- 1 egg

- 3 tbsp milk (3.5% fat)

- icing sugar made from erythritol for rolling

Preparation steps

1. Cut the chocolate roughly and melt it over a hot and uncooked bath of water. Split the vanilla pod longitudinally and remove the pulp.

2. Mix pulp, flour, cacao, baked powder, and salt with the mixture. Mix butter, sweetheart, egg, and milk in pieces. Put in chocolate that has been melted. Knead all in a smooth shortcut pastry quickly. Wrap for 2 hours in the fastening movie and chill.

3. Remove the dough, slightly flatten, from small portions, and shape into balls. Place the top on a baker sheet lined with baking paper and roll it in powdered sugar. Bake for about 8 minutes in a pre-heated oven, 180 ° C (150 ° C convector; 2-3 level gas). The cookies on the outside should be tight and on the inside juicy. Take off the wire rack and let it cool.

Banana Chocolate Cake

Preparation: 20 min Ready in 1 h

Ingredients

- 250 g flour

- 250 ml soy drink (soy milk)

- 100 g sugar

- 80 ml of oil

- 2 tbsp soy flour

- 4 tbsp water

- 1 pack baking powder

- 3 tbsp dark cocoa powder

- 2 bananas

Preparation steps

1. Preheat the oven to 180 ° C, grease the loaf pan with oil to cool.

2. Put all dry ingredients in a bowl, stir all wet ingredients together. Mix in the dry ingredients quickly. Peel the bananas, halve lengthways and cut into pieces, fold in.

3. Distribute the dough evenly in the loaf pan, smooth it out and bake for about 30-40 minutes (do a stick test). Let cool down a little, turn out of the mould onto a plate and let cool down completely. Cut into slices and serve with coffee.

Low Carb Hazelnut Macaroons

Preparation: 20 min Ready in 40 min

Ingredients

- 3 eggs

- 1 tsp lemon juice

- 100 g fine birch sugar powder (xylitol)

- ½ vanilla pod

- 250 g ground hazelnut kernels

- ½ tsp cinnamon

Preparation steps

1. Separate eggs (use egg yolks otherwise). Beat the egg whites with lemon juice in a bowl with the whisk of the hand mixer until frothy, gradually pour in the xylitol, and beat the mixture until it has tips.

2. Halve the vanilla pod lengthways and scrape out the pulp with a knife. Mix the hazelnuts with the vanilla pulp and cinnamon and fold into the whipped cream.

3. Pour the mixture into a piping bag with a large perforated nozzle and squirt small dots onto a baking sheet lined with baking paper. Bake in a preheated oven at 160 ° C (convection 140 ° C; gas: setting 1–2) for 15–20 minutes.

4. Take out, remove from the baking sheet with the baking paper, and let cool down.

Sweet Pretzels

Preparation: 40 min

Ready in 1 h 25 min

Ingredients

- 200 g spelled flour type 1050

- 50 g ground hazelnuts

- 50 g whole cane sugar

- 1 pinch vanilla powder

- ¼ organic lemon

- 1 pinch salt

- 100 g butter

- 2 eggs

- 1 egg yolk

- 1 tbsp milk (3.5% fat)

- 1 tbsp raw cane sugar

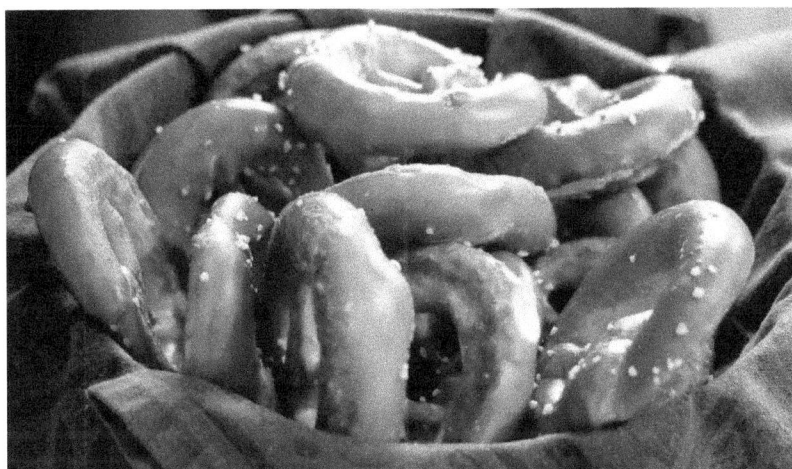

Preparation steps

1. For the dough, mix the flour with nuts, whole cane sugar, vanilla powder, grated lemon zest, and salt in a mixing bowl. Chop in the butter with the dough card, add the eggs and quickly knead into a smooth dough. Cover the dough and let it cool for about 30 minutes.

2. Shape the dough into small pencil-sized rolls 15 cm long and twist into small pretzels. Place these on a baking sheet lined with baking paper.

3. To brush the egg yolk with the milk, whisk and brush the pretzels with it. Bake the biscuits until golden yellow for 10–15 minutes; turn them immediately in the sugar and leave to cool on a wire rack.

Chapter Four. Brownie

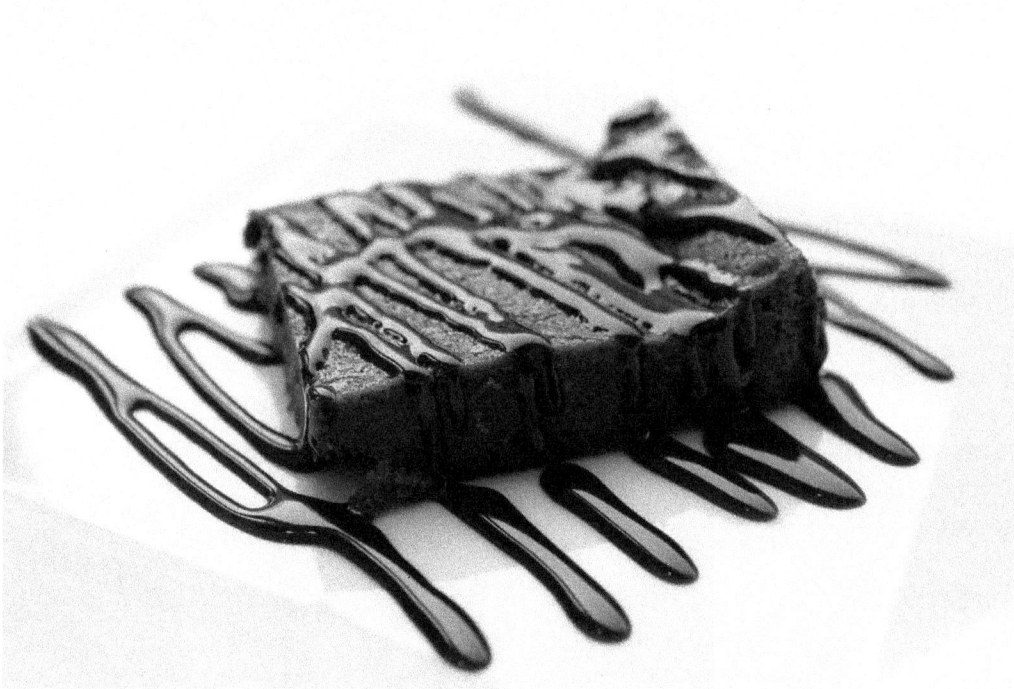

Sauerkraut brownies with blackberries

Preparation: 25 min

Ready in 1 h

Ingredients

- 100 g warm butter

- 120 g coconut blossom sugar

- 1 vanilla pod

- 200 g spelled flour

- 1 packet baking powder

- 100 g cocoa powder

- 1 pinch salt

- 3 eggs

- 300 ml milk

- 160 g wine sauerkraut

- 125 g blackberry

- 4 tbsp almond sticks

Preparation steps

1. Beat the blossom sugar butter and cocoa until it is creamy. Scrape out the pulp and half the vanilla pud along with the pulp. Flour, baking powder, cocoa, salt, eggs, and milk in a whisk of vanilla pulp.

2. Rinse the sauerkraut in hot water, thoroughly squeeze out and cut into tiny parts. Remove the mixture of the coconut butter and almond sticks into the batter.

3. Wash the blackberries and drain them. In a baking platter with baked paper, press the blackberries and bake for 30 to 35 minutes (stick test), in a preheated fire oven at 180 ° C (fan oven 160 ° C; gas at level 2 to 3).

4. Cool and serve the brownie sauerkraut and blackberries.

Sweet Potato Brownies

Preparation: 50 min

Ready in 1 h 40 min

Ingredients

- 600 g sweet potatoes

- 15 dates

- 4 tbsp coconut oil (melted)

- 5 tbsp honey

- 100 g wholemeal spelled flour

- 100 g ground almond

- ½ tsp salt

- 8 tbsp cocoa powder

- 2 tbsp almond butter

Preparation steps

1. Wash, peel, and cut the sweet potatoes into large pieces. Put this in a saucepan with some water and cook for about 20 minutes until the sweet potato is soft.

2. Put the soft sweet potato pieces together with the pitted dates in a food processor and puree to a paste.

3. Mix 2 tablespoons of coconut oil, 4 tablespoons of honey, wholegrain spelled flour, ground almonds, salt and 6 tablespoons of cocoa powder in a large bowl, and knead thoroughly with the sweet potato and date mix. Pour the finished dough into a 26 x 20-centimetre mould lined with baking paper and bake in a preheated oven at 180 ° C (convection: 160 ° C; gas: level 2–3) for about 50 minutes.

4. If no batter sticks to the wooden stick when you pierce the sweet potato brownie, it is ready and can be taken out of the oven. Now the whole thing has to cool for about 15 minutes so that the brownie doesn't fall apart when you lift it out.

5. For the glaze, melt 1 tbsp honey, 2 tbsp coconut oil, 2 tbsp almond butter, and 2 tbsp cocoa powder in a small saucepan and stir together. Then cool down to room temperature, for example, in the refrigerator.

6. Before the sweet potato brownie can be glazed, it must be completely cooled—otherwise, the glaze will melt! Then divide the sweet potato brownies into 16 pieces and serve.

Raspberry Brownies

Ingredients

- 150 g dark chocolate

- 250 g butter

- 5 eggs

- 100 g raw cane sugar

- 1 tsp vanilla powder

- 180 g spelled flour type 630

- 3 tbsp cocoa powder

- 1 tsp baking powder

- 400 g raspberries

Preparation steps

1. Roughly chop the chocolate with a knife. Melt the butter with the chocolate over a hot water bath and then let it cool down slightly. Mix the eggs with the whole cane sugar and vanilla powder in a bowl until creamy white. Add the chocolate butter and stir in. Mix the flour with the cocoa and baking powder and stir into the chocolate mixture. Pour about half of the dough onto the baking sheet lined with baking paper (or in a baking pan) and spread it on top. Sprinkle the selected raspberries on top and smooth the rest of the batter over it.

2. Bake for about 15 – 20 minutes in a preheated oven (fan oven: 160 ° C; gas: level 2–3) to keep the pulver moist. Then pick it up and let it get cool. Cut into pieces and, if you like, serve powdered sugar.

Brownie Cheesecake

Preparation: 30 min

Ready in 1 h

Ingredients

- 100 g dark chocolate (70% cocoa content)

- 125 g room temperature butter

- 100 g raw cane sugar

- 3 eggs

- 300 g quark (20% fat)

- 125 g spelled flour type 1050

- ½ packet baking powder

- ½ tsp vanilla powder

- 1 pinch salt

Preparation steps

1. For the chocolate mass, roughly chop the chocolate over a hot, non-boiling water bath. Then let cool down a little.

2. Mix the butter with the raw cane sugar in a bowl until creamy. Stir in the eggs and quark. Mix the flour with baking powder, vanilla, and salt and stir the flour mixture into the batter. Divide the dough and stir in the chocolate under half.

3. Fill the baking tin alternately in 3–4 layers and carefully marble with a fork. Bake in a preheated oven at 180 ° C (convection 160 ° C; gas: level 2–3) for 30 minutes. Take out and let cool on a wire rack. Cut into pieces for serving.

Zucchini-Brownies

Preparation: 30 min ready in 55 min

Ingredients

- 350 g zucchini

- 60 g coconut oil

- 50 g dark chocolate (70% cocoa content)

- 100 g wholemeal spelled flour

- 100 g spelled flour (type 630)

- 80 g coconut blossom sugar

- 50 g cocoa powder

- 1 tsp baking powder

- ½ tsp vanilla powder

- 1 pinch salt

- 2 eggs

Preparation steps

1. Wash and grate the zucchini. Put in a sieve and squeeze out some liquid. Melt coconut oil in a small saucepan over low heat. Roughly chop the chocolate.

2. Put flours, coconut blossom sugar, cocoa powder, baking powder, vanilla powder, salt, eggs, and liquid coconut oil in a bowl. Process all ingredients with the whisk of a hand mixer to smooth dough. Mix in the zucchini well, fold in the chocolate.

3. Pour the dough into a pan lined with baking paper and smooth it out. Bake in a preheated oven at 180 ° C (convection 160 ° C; gas: level 2–3) for 20–25 minutes (stick test). Then let cool completely in the mold. Cut into pieces and enjoy.

Bean brownies

Preparation: 20 min ready in 1 h

Ingredients

For the bean brownies

- 20th soft dates (soaked in hot water for 10 minutes)

- 180 g kidney beans (drained weight; can)

- 120 ml rapeseed oil

- 130 ml almond drink (almond milk) (or other vegetable milk)

- 3 eggs

- 50 g delicate oat flakes

- 50 g ground almond kernels

- 50 g cocoa powder

- 1 tsp baking powder

- 1 pinch salt

- 5 tbsp chopped walnut kernels

For the frosting

- 1 ripe avocado

- 3 tbsp coconut oil (melted)

- 3 tbsp espresso

- 3 tbsp cocoa powder

- 5 tbsp maple syrup

- streusel or coarse sea salt as desired

Preparation steps

1. Puree the dates and kidney beans in a blender, food processor, or with a hand blender to a creamy purée.

2. Add rapeseed oil, almond drink, eggs, oat flakes, ground almonds, cocoa powder, baking powder, and salt to the date and bean puree and stir to make a brownie batter.

3. Fold the chopped walnuts into the dough and pour the dough into a baking dish (approx. 26 x 20 centimeters) lined with baking paper. Bake in a preheated oven at 180 ° C (convection 160 ° C; gas: level 2–3) for about 30 minutes. Then let it cool down completely.

4. Now process all the ingredients for the frosting with a hand blender or a food processor into a fine chocolate cream and use a spatula to spread over the bean brownie. Refine with toppings as desired, cut into 16 pieces, and store in the refrigerator.

Luscious Walnut Chocolate Brownies

Preparation: 30 min ready in 55 min

Ingredients

- 180 g pitted dates

- 30 ml water

- 6 tbsp salted butter

- 210 g chopped dark chocolate

- 2 eggs (l)

- 2 tbsp cocoa powder

- 2 tbsp wholemeal spelled flour

- 130 g california walnuts (roughly chopped)

- 2 tbsp powdered sugar

Preparation steps

1. Preheat the oven to 180 degrees (gas: level 2, convection: 160 degrees). Grease a rectangular baking pan (23 cm) and line it with baking paper.

2. Put dates and water in a blender and puree to a paste. Put aside.

3. Melt the butter and chocolate in a large pan while stirring. Take the pan off the heat, let the chocolate cool down a bit and then stir in the date paste. Then gradually stir in the eggs carefully. Sift the cocoa and flour into a bowl, then add to the pan and mix with a wooden spoon to form a smooth batter.

4. Add walnuts to the dough, mix in and then pour the dough into the prepared baking pan. Then bake for 20 to 25 minutes until the brownie batter is firm in the middle. Then let cool down completely. Then decorate with a little icing sugar and a stencil (e.g. cappuccino stencils) with Christmas motifs.

Gluten-free Chocolate Cake

Preparation: 40 min

Ingredients

- 200 g dark chocolate couverture (gluten-free)

- 200 g butter

- 150 g whole cane sugar

- 5 eggs

- 100 g ground almond

- 2 tsp baking powder

- 250 g potato starch

- 250 g cornmeal

- 40 g cocoa powder

Preparation steps

1. Roughly chop the couverture with a knife. Melt over a hot water bath and allow cooling.

2. Mix butter with sugar in a bowl until frothy. Gradually stir in eggs until a creamy mixture is formed. Stir liquid chocolate, almonds, baking powder, starch, cornflour, and cocoa into the foam mixture.

3. Line the baking sheet with parchment paper. Spread the dough on the baking sheet and bake in the preheated oven at 180 ° C (convection 160 ° C; gas: level 2–3) for about 25–30 minutes. Make a chopstick test.

Brownies with Nuts

Preparation: 30 min

Ingredients

- 250 g soft butter

- 150 g sugar

- 4 eggs

- 200 g dark chocolate

- 250 g ground hazelnuts

- 250 g flour

- ½ tsp baking powder

- ½ tsp cinnamon

- 1 tbsp cocoa powder

For covering

- 250 g butter

- 250 g sugar

- 800 g condensed milk

- 120 g honey

- 600 g mixed nuts e.g. b. (hazelnuts, pistachios, almonds, walnuts, etc

Preparation steps

1. Preheat the oven to 200 ° C top and bottom heat.

2. Mix the butter with the sugar and the eggs until creamy. Grate the chocolate and stir into the butter-egg mixture with the ground nuts, flour, baking powder, cinnamon, and cocoa. Spread the dough about 2 cm thick on a greased baking sheet and bake in the preheated oven for 20-25 minutes. For the topping, heat the butter, add the sugar and condensed milk, mix in the honey, bring to a boil and simmer for 5-10 minutes, stirring, until everything is caramelized. Fold in the coarsely chopped, mixed nuts, pour over the finished brownie batter, spread on, and let cool. Serve cut into small rectangles.

Halloween Brownies

Preparation: 30 min ready in 1 h 40 min

Ingredients

- 600 g hokkaido pumpkin

- 75 g whole cane sugar

- 1 tsp cinnamon powder

- ½ tsp ginger powder

- 1 pinch ground mace

- 200 g dark chocolate (at least 70% cocoa content)

- 90 g agave syrup

- ½ tsp vanilla powder

- 175 g room temperature butter

- 1 pinch salt

- 5 eggs

- 100 g spelled flour type 1050

- 1 tbsp baking powder

- 50 g cocoa powder

- 200 g cream cheese (40% fat in dry matter)

Preparation steps

1. Cut the calf, cut half, centre, and wedge the pulp. In a bakery boiler with a bakery, cover the pumpkin and baker for about 40 minutes in a preheated oven at 200 ° C (fan oven: 180 ° C, gas level 3).

2. Take the kitchen, fine puree, cinnamon, ginger, and mace, all with whole cane sugar, and allow to cool.

3. Cut the chocolate roughly into it and melt it over a bath of hot water.

4. Mix agave powder, butter, and salt in the mixture with agave syrup to creamy. Remove in 3 eggs one by one. Chocolate subject. Mix meal, baking powder, and cocoa powder and then add chocolate and agave syrup carefully. In the mould, add the mixture and smooth.

5. With cream cheese, mix the pumpkin puree and the rest of the eggs. Put into the mould the mixture of the pumpkin and cream cheese and sprinkle it onto the chocolate with a wood spoon.

6. Bake for 30–35 minutes in the oven at 200 degrees C (fan oven 180 degrees C, gas level 3). Take it out, let it cool, cut it in pieces.

Raw Brownies with Cashew Nuts

Ingredients

- 450 g dried dates

- 150 g cashew nuts

- 300 g ground almond kernels

- 110 g cocoa powder (heavily de-oiled)

- 45 g almond flour (3 tbsp)

- 1 pinch salt

- ½ vanilla pod

Preparation steps

1. Just cover the dates with water and leave to soak overnight. On the next day, pour off the date water, put it on top, and set aside. Puree the softened dates with a hand blender to a creamy paste and add some date water if necessary, so that the mixture becomes creamy.

2. Chop the cashew nuts. Halve the vanilla pod lengthways, scrape out the pulp. Mix the almonds, cocoa, almond flour, 100 g cashew nuts, 1 pinch of salt, and vanilla pulp in a bowl, and knead with the date paste.

3. Pour the dough into a baking dish or baking tin (30 x 20 cm) lined with baking paper and press firmly.

4. Let the dough set in the refrigerator for at least 4 hours. Then cut into 15 pieces and decorate with the remaining cashew nuts.

Vegan Brownies with Black Beans

Preparation: 20 min

Ready in 45 min

Ingredients

- 400 g black beans (glass or can)

- 70 g oatmeal

- 2 tsp espresso

- 70 g virgin coconut oil

- 130 g agave syrup

- 200 g vegan dark chocolate (at least 70% cocoa)

- 1 tsp tartar baking powder

- 1 pinch salt

- ½ tsp vanilla powder

Preparation steps

1. Put the beans in a colander and drain.

2. Grind the oatmeal into a coarse flour in a powerful mixer.

3. Heat coconut oil over a water bath so that it becomes liquid.

4. Chop the chocolate and add 130 g together with the beans, espresso, coconut oil, agave syrup, baking powder, salt, and vanilla powder in the mixer and process into a creamy dough. Fold in half of the remaining chocolate.

5. Line a baking sheet with parchment paper. Pour in the batter, smooth it out and sprinkle with the remaining chocolate. Bake vegan brownies at 175 ° C (fan 150 ° C; gas: level 2) for about 15–20 minutes.

6. Allow to cool after baking, remove from mold, and cut into pieces before serving.

Pecan Chocolate Cake

Preparation: 25 min ready in 55 min

Ingredients

- 200 g dark chocolate (70% cocoa content)

- 100 g milk chocolate with 30% cocoa content

- 110 g butter

- 3 tsp creme fraiche cheese

- 130 g pecans

- 3 eggs

- 100 g whole cane sugar

- ½ tsp salt

- 180 g wheat flour type 1050

- 10 g baking powder

Preparation steps

1. Roughly chop both chocolates and melt them with butter over a hot water bath. Stir in the crème fraîche.

2. Line a baking pan or a small deep baking sheet with parchment paper.

3. Roughly chop the nuts. In a bowl, whip the eggs with sugar and salt until the sugar has dissolved. Gradually stir the cooled chocolate into the egg mix. Mix the flour with the nuts and baking powder and stir in as well.

4. Pour the batter into the baking pan and smooth it out. Bake the cake in a preheated oven at 180 ° C (convection 160 ° C; gas: level 2–3) for about 25–30 minutes—it should still be a little soft in the middle so that a little dough can stick to the stick test. Let cool and cut into pieces (approx. 5 x 6 cm).

Brownies with Almonds

Preparation: 1 h

Ingredients

- 100 g dark chocolate
- 125 g soft butter
- 150 g brown sugar
- 2 eggs
- 100 g flour
- ½ tsp baking powder
- salt
- 1 tsp real bourbon vanilla
- 150 g almond sticks
- fat for the baking pan
- icing sugar for dusting

Preparation steps

1. Chop the chocolate, chop and stir frequently and then put aside in a double boiler. In a bowl with a hand mixer, mix the butter and brown sugar until creamy. Remove the eggs and add the chocolate liquid. Top/bottom heat preheat the oven to 200 ° C.

2. Mix flour, salt, and vanilla with baking powder. Remove the almonds into the dough with the flour blend. Fat the baker's pot. In the mould, put the dough into the oven for approximately 30-40 minutes, until a stick inserted in the middle comes out smoothly. Fall

on a grid and allow it to fully cool down. To be served, dust and cut into pieces with powdered sugar.

Sauerkraut Brownies with Raspberries

Ingredients

- 100 g warm butter

- 120 g coconut blossom sugar

- 1 vanilla pod

- 200 g spelled flour

- 1 packet baking powder

- 100 g cocoa powder

- 1 pinch

- salt

- 3 eggs

- 300 ml milk

- 160 g wine sauerkraut

- 125 g raspberry

- 4 tbsp almond sticks

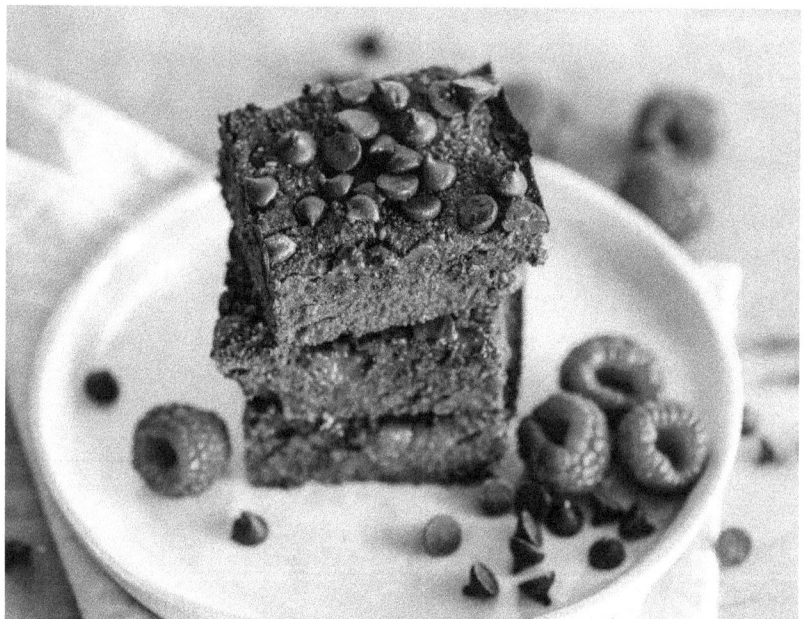

Preparation steps

1. Beat the butter and coconut blossom sugar until creamy. Halve the vanilla pod lengthways and scrape out the pulp. Whisk the vanilla pulp with the flour, baking powder, cocoa, salt, eggs, and milk.

2. Rinse the sauerkraut under hot water, squeeze out thoroughly and cut into small pieces. Stir into the batter with the butter coconut blossom sugar mixture and almond sticks.

3. Wash and drain the raspberries. Put the dough in a baking dish lined with baking paper, press in the raspberries, and bake in a preheated oven at 180 ° C (fan oven 160 ° C; gas: level 2–3) for 30–35 minutes (stick test).

4. Let the sauerkraut brownies with raspberries cool and serve.

Brownie Strawberry Cake

Preparation: 45 min

Ingredients

- 200 g dark chocolate
- 100 g butter
- 2 tsp instant espresso powder
- 2 tbsp sugar
- 2 eggs (size l)
- 4 tbsp flour
- 300 g whipped cream
- 1 pack vanilla sugar
- 2 pack cream stiffener
- 1 pinch cinnamon
- 300 g strawberries

Preparation steps

1. Preheat the oven to 180° C. Melt the chocolate over a hot water bath with 2 teaspoons of water. Add the butter, let it melt, and stir in.

2. Mix the espresso powder with 1 tablespoon of hot water and mix with the sugar into the chocolate mass. Stir vigorously for 5 minutes until the sugar has completely dissolved.

3. Remove the bowl from the water bath and let cool down a little (at least 5 minutes). In a second bowl, beat the eggs until they are white and frothy. Fold in the flour and the still liquid chocolate mixture.

4. Draw 2 circles approx. 20-24 cm in size on baking paper, turn the baking paper upside down on the baking sheet and spread the dough on the circles

5. Bake in the oven (middle rack) for about 20 minutes, until you can pull out a pricked wooden stick.

6. Take out of the oven and let cool down. Beat the cream with the cream stabilizer and vanilla sugar until stiff. Wash, clean, lay the strawberries, cut them smaller if necessary.

7. Spread half of the sahs on one base, cover with strawberries, place the second base on top and garnish with cream and strawberries, serve dusted with cinnamon.

8. Let cool down briefly in the tin, then turn out and serve warm with whipped cream or 1 small scoop of vanilla ice cream.

Brownie with Cherries

Preparation: 30 min

Ready in 50 min

Ingredients

- 200 g chocolate (70% cocoa content)

- 200 g butter

- 4 eggs

- 200 g sugar

- 100 g flour

- 1 glass morello cherries

- 1 tbsp. potato starch

- 1 pinch cinnamon

- 1 tsp. sugar

- butter for the mold

Preparation steps

1. Preheat the oven to 210 °. Grease a baking pan 24 cm in diameter.

2. Melt the chocolate over a hot water bath, take it off the stove and stir in the cold butter little by little. Stir the mixture until creamy. Separate the eggs. Beat the egg white until stiff, then

beat the egg yolks with the sugar until frothy until the mixture turns white and creamy. Carefully stir into the cooled chocolate and butter mixture. Fold in the egg whites. Sift the flour over it and fold it carefully. Put the dough in the greased baking pan and place on the middle rack for 20 minutes

3. For the cherry sauce, put the cherries and the liquid (except for 3 tablespoons) in a saucepan, heat with sugar. Put the cinnamon, starch, and the 3 tablespoons of juice in a cup and stir until smooth. Add the mixed starch to the cherries while stirring, bring to the boil, and set aside.

4. Cut the cake into 15 squares and then into triangles. Arrange two triangles with the cherry sauce on plates and serve.

Coffee-Chocolate Cake

Preparation: 25 min ready in 1 h

Ingredients

- 150 g dark chocolate 70% cocoa content

- 100 g milk chocolate with 30% cocoa content

- 100 g soft butter

- 2 tsp crème fraîche at least 30% fat

- 100 g almond kernels

- 3 eggs

- 200 g brown sugar

- ½ tsp salt

- 180 g flour

- 10 g cocoa powder

- 10 g baking powder

- 1 tbsp rum

- 20 g instant coffee

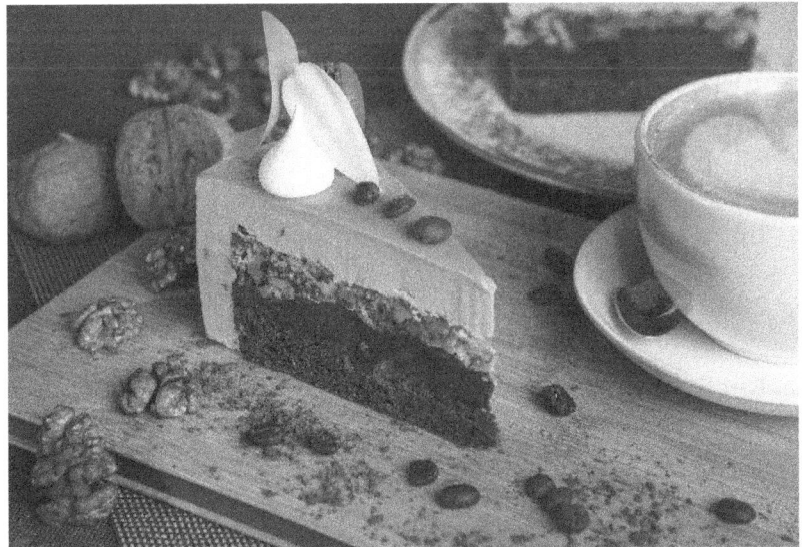

Preparation steps

1. Chop both kinds of chocolate roughly and melt it over a hot water bath together with butter. Slowly cool, then stir in the fresh cream. To 180 ° C (top and lower heat) pre-heat oven. Line a parchment paper baking sheet. Cut the almonds very hard. In a bowl, add the sugar and salt to the eggs until the sugar is dissolved. Mix in the chocolate-butter blend gradually. Stir. Mix the meal and the baked powder with the cocoa and sieve. Warm down the rum, dissolve the coffee in it and add the meal and almonds to the dough. Place and smooth the dough on the baker. Bake brownies for 35-40 minutes in a hot oven on the center rack (test the stick!). Allow the brownies to cool down and chop (about.

2. Wash the orange with hot water for garnishing, rub it dry and remove the peel with fine zest. Half the fruit, squeeze the juice, and then enter into a small cup of sugar. Additionally, add sugar and reduce to syrup the mixture. Add the orange zest and allow it to dry until the syrup has a golden brown color.

Brownies with Coffee

Ingredients

- 350 g dark couverture

- 200 g chopped walnut kernels

- 6 eggs

- 300 g sugar

- scraped pulp of a vanilla pod

- 1 pinch salt

- 200 ml oil

- 150 g flour

- 3 tbsp cocoa powder

- 2 tsp baking powder

- 100 ml espresso

- powdered sugar

Preparation steps

1. Coarsely chop 100 g couverture. Crush the remaining couverture and melt it in a bowl in a hot water bath. Mix eggs with sugar, vanilla pulp, and salt until frothy. Add oil and stir briefly until smooth.

2. Mix the flour, cocoa, and baking powder and fold carefully into the batter. Finally, fold the melted couverture, chopped walnuts, and chopped couverture with half of the espresso into the batter.

3. Place the dough on a baking sheet (30 x 20 cm) lined with baking paper and smooth it out. Bake in the preheated oven (180 ° top and bottom heat, middle rack) for about 30 minutes.

4. Take out and let cool slightly. Then spread the rest of the espresso on the still-warm cake and let it cool down. Cut into pieces for serving and dust with powdered sugar.

Brownies with Mixed Nuts

Preparation: 35 min

Ready in 1 h 10 min

Ingredients

- 150 g butter

- 2 eggs

- 125 g flour

- ½ tsp baking powder

- 35 g cocoa powder

- 200 g sugar

- 1 tbsp vanilla sugar

- 125 g dark chocolate drops

- 60 g pistachio nuts

- 60 g dried cranberries

- 1 handful peeled almond kernels

Preparation steps

1. Preheat the oven to 160 ° C top and bottom heat and line the baking pan with baking paper.

2. Melt the butter in a small saucepan, then let it cool for about 10 minutes. Whisk the eggs well and stir in the butter.

3. Sieve the flour, baking powder, and cocoa. Add the sugar, vanilla sugar, chocolate chips, pistachios, and cranberries and mix in briefly.

4. Pour into the form, smooth it out and sprinkle with the almonds. Bake in the oven for 30-35 minutes. Let cool and serve cut into pieces.

Chapter Five. Bars

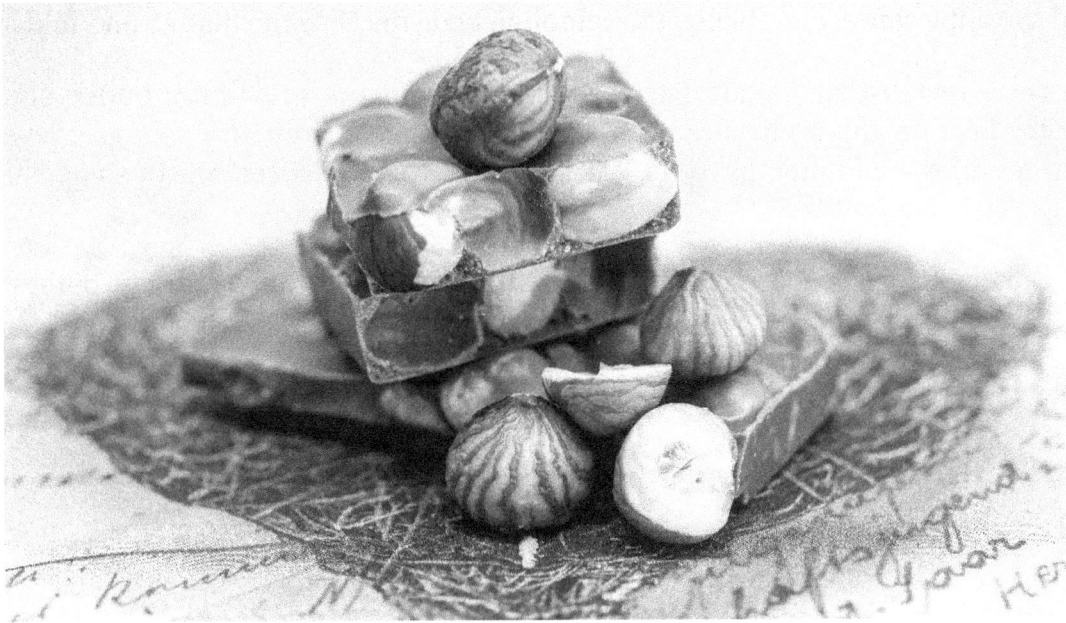

Moist Cheesecake Bars

Preparation: 10 min ready in 1 h

Ingredients

- 60 g butter

- 80 g sugar

- 1 packet vanilla sugar

- 2 eggs

- 500 g low-fat quark

- 300 g applesauce (without sugar)

- 125 g wheat semolina

- 50 g dried mango

Preparation steps

1. Put 50 g butter, sugar, vanilla sugar, and the eggs in a bowl and add the quark spoon by spoon. Mix briefly but thoroughly with the hand mixer.

2. Add the applesauce, and finally, the semolina and stir. Dice the mango and fold in.

3. Grease a rectangular baking pan (20x30 cm) with the remaining butter and fill in the dough. Bake in the preheated oven at 180 ° C (convection: 160 ° C, gas: level 2) for 40 minutes on the middle rack. If the cake turns too brown, cover it with some aluminum foil for the last 10 minutes.

4. Let the cheesecake cool a little in the mold. Halve lengthways and cut both strips into 6 pieces about 5x10 cm. Wrap in foil to take away.

Coconut Papaya Bars

Preparation: 25 min

Ingredients

- 150 ml coconut milk
- 2 tbsp agave syrup
- 75 g coconut oil (5 tbsp)
- 1 tsp turmeric powder
- 1 papaya
- 300 g desiccated coconut
- 400 g dark chocolate (at least 70% cocoa content)

Preparation steps

1. Put coconut milk with agave syrup, coconut oil, and turmeric in a saucepan and heat over low heat for about 5 minutes, stirring occasionally. Then take it off the stove.

2. In the meantime, peel and core the papaya and cut into pieces. Puree the papaya pulp with a hand blender.

3. Mix the papaya puree and desiccated coconut with the coconut milk, place in a flat baking dish lined with baking paper, and place in the freezer for 2–3 hours.

4. Shortly before the end of the freezing time, melt the chocolate in a water bath. Remove the coconut papaya mixture from the freezer and cut into 20 bars. Cover coconut and mango bars with chocolate and chill for at least 30 minutes before serving.

Walnut Chocolate Bars

Preparation: 40 min

Ready in 1 h 30 min

Ingredients

- 200 g flour

- 50 g food starch

- 200 g ground almond kernels

- 2 tsp baking powder

- 1 pinch salt

- 150 g sugar

- 1 egg

- 250 g yoghurt butter (cold)

- 250 g dark chocolate couverture

- 250 dark chocolate couverture

- 200 g walnut kernels

Preparation steps

1. Mix the flour with the starch, almonds, baking powder, a pinch of salt and sugar, and pile on the work surface. Make a well in the middle, add the egg.

2. Cut the butter into pieces, spread around the flour. Chop everything from the outside in with a large knife until you get crumbs. Then knead quickly with your hands to form a smooth dough, add 1–2 tablespoons of water as required.

3. Wrap the dough in cling film and place in the refrigerator for at least 30 minutes.

4. Divide the dough into 50 pieces and shape into rolls. Line a baking sheet with parchment paper. Spread the rolls of dough spaced apart on the baking sheet and bake in a preheated oven at 180 ° C (fan oven 160 ° C; gas: level 2–3) for about 15 minutes until light brown.

5. Remove the bar and allow cooling on a wire rack.

6. Chop the couverture, melt over a hot water bath. In the meantime, coarsely chop walnuts and roast them until golden brown in a pan without fat.

7. Coat bars with chocolate, roll in walnuts, and let dry on a wire rack.

Granola Bars

Preparation: 40 min

Ingredients

- 160 g mixed seeds (flax seeds, sunflower seeds, hemp seeds, pumpkin seeds)

- 120 g almond kernels

- 60 g pistachios

- 60 g oatmeal

- 40 g raisins (sugar-free and sulfur-free)

- 40 g dried cranberries (sugar-free and sulfur-free)

- 80 g maple syrup

- 70 g almond butter

- 50 g coconut oil

- 30 g cocoa nibs (3 tbsp)

- 1 pinch salt

Preparation steps

1. Chop the seeds and kernels into small pieces. Spread this with the oat flakes on a baking sheet and roast in a preheated oven at 200 ° C (convection 180 ° C; gas: level 3) for about 10 minutes. Then take it out of the oven and let it cool down for 10 minutes.

2. Then let coconut oil melt in a small saucepan for 2 minutes over low heat. Then put all the ingredients in a bowl and mix well. Line a baking dish (25 x 35 cm) with baking paper, pour the granola mixture into the dish, and spread it with a spoon.

3. Cover the mixture with cling film and press firmly into the mould with your hands. Place the mould in the freezer for 1 hour. Then cut the cold and firm mixture into bars and serve. To keep them fresh, keep the bars in the refrigerator or freezer.

Cheesecake with a Biscuit Base

Preparation: 40 min

Ready in 1 h 20 min

Ingredients

- 150 g whole grain biscuit

- 50 g butter

- 1 tbsp beet syrup

- 500 g ricotta

- 300 g low-fat quark

- 2 eggs

- 2 tbsp food starch

- ½ tsp vanilla powder

- 50 g raw cane sugar

- 100 g chopped almond

- 150 g small candy bars

- 150 ml whipped cream

Preparation steps

1. In a clean tea towel, place the biscuits and use the rolling pine for crumbling. Melt the butter and sugar beet syrup in a small casserole over low heats and mix. Line the bakery paper in the spring shape pot. Pour the mixture into the biscuit and squeeze it down.

2. Mix the quark with the ricotta. Add egg, whisk, vanilla powder, and sugar to the macerated starch gradually. Fold in the cream of the almonds. Put the chocolate bars on the bottom of the cake and smooth over it. In a pre-heated oven, cook for 50-60 minutes at 180 ° C (convection 160 ° C; gas: 2-3)

3. Taken out of the oven, let the cheesecake cool in the pot for a while. Remove from the mould the cheesecake and leave to cool completely.

4. Shake the cream into the steepness and serve the cake.

Oatmeal and Nut Bars

Preparation: 45 min

Ready in 1 h 5 min

Ingredients

- 50 g banana chips

- 70 g dried fig

- 200 g honey

- 140 g cane sugar

- 100 g oatmeal

- 2 tsp potash

- ½ tsp cinnamon

- 220 g spelled flour

- 1 tsp tartar baking powder

Preparation steps

1. Put the banana chips in a blender with a knife and chop. Remove the hard stalks from the figs and cut the flesh into small pieces. Put the honey and sugar in a saucepan, heat slowly over a low temperature until the sugar has dissolved. Add the oatmeal, banana chips, and figs, and simmer for 2-3 minutes.

2. Set aside and let cool.

3. Preheat the oven to 180 ° C top and bottom heat.

4. Stir the potash in a little water until smooth. Mix the flour with the cinnamon, baking powder, and the potash into the oatmeal mixture. Place on the lightly floured work surface and knead. Roll out the dough approx. 1 cm thick and place on a baking sheet lined with baking paper. Bake in the preheated oven for about 20 minutes. Then heat the honey, cut the warm dough sheet into rectangles, brush them with the honey and decorate with oat flakes and almonds or macadamia nuts. Let it cool down and keep it dry.

Muesli Bars with Chocolate

Preparation: 30 min

Ingredients

- 160 g butter

- 240 g honey

- 140 g mixed dried fruit e.g. b. apricots, apples, figs, plums, etc.

- 120 g ground almond kernels

- 80 g ground hazelnuts

- 70 g coarsely chopped hazelnuts

- 70 g desiccated coconut

- 180 g cereal flakes z. b. oats, barley, wheat, rye and spelled

- 3 tbsp flour

- 200 g dark chocolate couverture

Preparation steps

1. Preheat the oven to 160 ° C top and bottom heat. Melt the butter with the honey in a saucepan over a low flame. Roughly chop the fruits and stir into the butter mixture with the almonds, nuts, desiccated coconut, flakes, and flour, spread 1 cm thick on a baking sheet lined with baking paper (30x24 cm), and bake in the oven for 30-35 minutes.

2. In the meantime, roughly chop the couverture and melt it over a hot, non-boiling water bath. Remove the liquid couverture from the water bath and let it cool slightly.

3. Take the finished muesli mixture out of the oven, let it cool, and cut into bars of 2x8 cm. Dip one side of this into the liquid chocolate and let it dry upside down on a wire rack or baking sheet.

Apricot and Coconut Bars

Preparation: 15 minutes

Ingredients

- 100 g dried apricots
- 30 g butter (2 tbsp.)
- 50 g liquid honey
- 80 g whole cane sugar (4 tbsp.)
- ½ organic orange
- 100 g spelled flakes
- 50 g desiccated coconut
- 40 g chopped almond kernels (4 tbsp.)

Preparation steps

1. Dice the apricots.

2. Put butter, honey, and sugar in a small saucepan and bring to the boil.

3. Rinse half an orange with hot water and rub dry. Rub 1 teaspoon of peel, squeeze out the juice.

4. Mix 1 tbsp. orange juice and zest spelled flakes, desiccated coconut, almonds, and diced apricots with the sweet butter.

5. Spread the mixture 1-1.5 cm thick with a damp rubber spatula on a baking sheet lined with baking paper. Bake in the preheated oven at 150 ° C (convection: 130 ° C, gas: level 1-2) on the middle rack for about 25 minutes. Let the plate cool down completely, then cut into bars.

Fig and Cranberry Bars

Preparation: 25 min

Ingredients

- 100 g walnut kernels
- 100 g dried fig
- 1 organic orange
- 80 g soft butter
- 100 g whole cane sugar
- 1 pinch salt
- 2 eggs
- 150 g whole wheat flour
- 2 tsp. tartar baking powder
- 100 g ground hazelnuts
- 100 g dried cranberries
- 1 tsp. cocoa powder
- ½ tsp. cardamom or cinnamon

Preparation steps

1. Grind the walnut kernels.
2. Finely dice the figs.
3. Rinse orange with hot water and rub dry. Finely grate the orange peel. Halve the fruit and squeeze out the juice.
4. Mix the butter, sugar, salt, and orange peel with the hand mixer. Stir in eggs.
5. Add flour, baking powder, figs, nuts, cranberries, cocoa, and cardamom and knead in.
6. Place the dough on a baking sheet lined with baking paper and roll it out under cling film.

7. Remove the foil and bake in a preheated oven at 180 ° C (convection: 160 ° C, gas: level 2–3) for about 30 minutes.

8. Drizzle the pastries with orange juice while they are still hot, let them steep for 5 minutes, then cut into bars and let cool on the work board.

Fruit Muesli Bars

Preparation: 20 min

Ready in 12 h 40 min

Ingredients

- 225 g fruit muesli (mixture without sugar)

- 50 g oatmeal

- 30 g butter

- 50 g whole cane sugar

- 100 g liquid honey

- 1 tsp apple juice

- 80 g rose hip pulp

Preparation steps

1. Mix the muesli and fleks.

2. Melt the butter in a pan. Add sugar, honey, and apple juice and bring to the boil while stirring. Cook over medium heat for 2 minutes, stirring, until the mixture is liquid and golden yellow.

3. Remove the pan from the heat, carefully stir in the muesli, and flecked mixture until it is evenly mixed.

4. Put the mixture on a baking sheet lined with baking paper, roll it out under cling film to a plate of approx. 25x20x1.5 cm.

5. Remove the foil and let the muesli mixture cool for at least 20 minutes.

6. Heat the rosehip puree and spread on the muesli block.

7. Cut the muesli blocks into bars and let them dry overnight on a work board.

Peanut Bars

Ingredients

- ½ orange
- 100 g unsalted peanut kernel
- 30 g butter
- 30 g whole cane sugar
- 100 g honey
- 150 g hearty oat flakes
- 50 g oatmeal
- 50 g raisins

Preparation steps

1. Squeeze the orange.
2. Roughly chop the peanuts.
3. Heat the butter, sugar, and honey in a saucepan until the sugar has melted.
4. Add 1 teaspoon of orange juice, oat flakes, oat flakes, and nuts and let them turn golden brown while stirring.
5. Stir in the raisins.
6. Spread the mixture on a baking sheet lined with baking paper with a damp rubber spatula and bake in the preheated oven at 150 ° C (fan oven 130 ° C, gas: level 1–2) on the middle rack for 10–15 mins.
7. Cut into bars while still warm, then let cool down completely.

Yoghurt Quark Layered Dish

Preparation: 10 min

Ingredients

- 40 g ladyfingers (6 ladyfingers)

- 2 tbsp passion fruit juice

- 75 g strawberries (6 strawberries)

- 2 tbsp yogurt (1.5% fat)

- 1 tbsp low-fat quark

- 2 half apricots (can)

- 1 tsp pistachios

- 1 tsp honey

Preparation steps

1. Spread the ladyfingers in a small flat bowl and drizzle evenly with the passion fruit juice.

2. Clean and wash the strawberries and put 1 nice berry aside. Cut the rest of the berries into small cubes and sprinkle over the ladyfingers.

3. In a small bowl, stir the yoghurt and quark until creamy. Distribute evenly on the strawberries.

4. Drain the apricot halves and cut into narrow wedges.

5. Roughly chop the pistachios.

6. Place the strawberry that was set aside in the middle of the layered dish and arrange the apricot wedges around it like flower petals. Sprinkle with pistachios, drizzle with honey and serve.

Caramel Pecan Cookies

Preparation: 40 min

Ingredients

- 250 g flour

- 1 tsp baking powder

- 1 pinch salt

- 200 g butter

- 225 g cane sugar

- 1 egg

- 50 g chopped pecans

- chocolate bar with caramel filling, (e.g. mars), diced into small pieces

Preparation steps

1. Preheat the oven to 180 ° C fan oven. Line 2 baking sheets with parchment paper.

2. Mix the flour with baking powder and salt. Whip soft butter with sugar until creamy; add egg, flour, nuts, and pieces of bars.

3. Shape the resulting mass into hazelnut-sized balls. Place the balls on the trays and press them flat.

4. Bake for about 15 minutes, remove and allow cooling on the trays, then removing from the trays and letting cool down completely. Store in a dry place.

Chocolate Bar with Caramel

Preparation: 50 min

Ready in 5 h 40 min

Ingredients

For the dough

- 300 g flour and flour to work with

- 100 g sugar

- 1 pinch salt

- 200 g butter

- 1 egg

- dried pulses for blind baking

For the caramel layer

- 600 ml whipped cream

- 300 g sugar

- 75 g butter

- 75 ml whiskey cream liqueur

- 400 g dark chocolate couverture

For the chocolate layer

- 400 g dark chocolate couverture

Preparation steps

1. Stack the meal on the surface of the job and make a middle hole. Spread on the edge of the meal, the sugar, salt, and Butter. Put the egg in the center and use a card to chop it all into crumbs. Knead with your hands to create smooth, hand-free dough. Wrap the film and put in the refrigerator for approximately 30 minutes.

2. Preheat the oven to 180 degrees centigrade. Line a deep parchment paper baker.

3. Fold off the dough to the height of a plate on a blurred work surface and place on the bakery plate. Several times, prick the bottom with a fork, cover the legumes and baking paper. In a hot oven, bake until golden 15-20 minutes. Remove the leguminous and paper and cool the base on the bakery plate.

4. Boil the cream, sugar, butter, and liqueur in a cup in the caramel layer while stirring for about 30 minutes over low heat, occasionally stirring, until golden yellow and thick. Remove from heat, mix the chocolate chopped and let it cool.

5. Smooth out the mixture on the floor. Allow it to cool down for approximately 2 hours.

6. To coat, chop the cover, melt and cool it again over a hot water bath. Lay on the caramel layer and set it for approximately 1 hour.

7. Serve in pieces. Serve.

Cream Slices with Raspberries

Preparation: 2 h 40 min

Ingredients

- 250 g raspberries

- 2 sheets gelatin

- 2 tbsp raspberry liqueur

- 150 g mascarpone

- 200 g whipped cream

- 3 tbsp cane sugar

- 1 packet vanilla sugar

- 1 packet cream stiffener

- 6 nut and granola bars

- lemon balm for garnish

Preparation steps

1. Wash and sort the berries. Approx. Puree 1/4 of it and strain through a sieve. Soak the gelatine in cold water. Then squeeze out and dissolve in warm liqueur. Stir into the puree.

2. Mix the mascarpone with the sugar and vanilla sugar until smooth, whip the cream with the cream stiffener until stiff and fold into the mascarpone, then stir in the raspberry puree.

3. Place the muesli bars with the long sides together and frame with aluminum foil (approx. 5 cm high). Spread 3/4 of the cream on the muesli platter, pour the raspberry puree on top, and spread the rest of the cream on top. Min. Chill for 2 hours. To serve, cut into 6 slices with a hot knife (dip briefly in hot water), garnish with the remaining berries and lemon balm.

Almond and Oatmeal Bars

Preparation: 15 minutes

Ready in 40 min

Ingredients

- 200 g dried fruit e.g. b. cherries and apricots

- 50 g raisins

- 50 g almond flakes

- 250 g tender oatmeal

- 100 g coarse-grain oatmeal

- 100 g coarse-grained spelled flakes

- 200 g brown cane sugar

- 50 g beet syrup

- 325 g butter

Preparation steps

1. Preheat the oven to 160 ° C fan oven.

2. Chop the dried fruit and mix with the raisins, almonds, oat, and spelled flakes, and cane sugar in a bowl. Slowly heat the sugar beet syrup and butter in a saucepan, stir and mix into the muesli mixture.

3. Spread the mixture evenly on a baking sheet lined with baking paper, approx. 1 cm thick.

4. Bake in the oven for 20-25 minutes until lightly golden brown. Take out of the oven, cut into approx. 5x10 cm long bars and leave to cool on a wire rack.

Layered Dish with Chocolate Bars

Preparation: 20 min

Ingredients

- 60 g ladyfingers

- 100 ml coffee

- 20 ml coffee liqueur

- 300 ml whipped cream at least 30% fat content

- 2 tbsp powdered sugar

- 1 tbsp vanilla sugar

- 100 g cream cheese

- 1 tbsp cocoa powder

- 1 chocolate bars z. b. mars

Preparation steps

1. Roughly break the ladyfingers and divide them into four glasses. Mix the cold coffee with the coffee liqueur and drizzle over the biscuits.

2. Beat the cream with the powdered sugar and vanilla sugar until stiff. Mix in the cocoa and cream cheese under half and layer over the ladyfingers.

3. Pour the rest of the cream over it and serve garnished with a sliced or finely chopped, ice-cold chocolate bar.

Chocolate Cakes

Preparation: 1 h

Ready in 1 h 25 min

Ingredients

For the cupcakes

- 200 g dark chocolate couverture

- 100 g butter

- 4 chocolate-caramel bars z. b. snickers

- 2 eggs

- 100 g sour cream

- 100 g sugar

- 250 g flour

- 2 tsp food starch

- 2 tsp baking powder

- 1 tbsp cocoa powder

- 1 pinch salt

For the topping

- 120 g soft butter

- 1 pinch vanilla pulp

- 60 g sugar

- 120 g cream cheese

- 1 tbsp caramel syrup

- 150 g powdered sugar

- 2 chocolate-caramel bars z. b. snickers

Preparation steps

1. Preheat the oven to 180 ° C fan oven. Grease a muffin tin and dust with flour.

2. Roughly chop the couverture. Heat the butter in a saucepan, add the couverture and let it melt while stirring. Let the mixture cool down a bit.

3. Cut the chocolate bars into 12 pieces approx. 2 cm in size.

4. Mix the eggs with the sour cream, sugar, and cooled chocolate butter. Mix the flour with the cornstarch, baking powder, cocoa, and salt. Stir the mixture into the egg and chocolate buttercream. Spread about two-thirds of the dough on the moulds and use a small spoon to form a hollow in the middle. Place a piece of a chocolate bar in each of the dough moulds and spread the rest of the dough over it. Bake the cupcakes on the middle rack for about 25 minutes. Then take it out and let it cool down.

5. For the topping, mix the butter, vanilla, and sugar until creamy, stir in the cream cheese, and caramel syrup. Now stir in enough powdered sugar until you have a sprayable mixture. Spread the cream on the cupcakes. Cut the chocolate and caramel bars into pieces and decorate the topping with them.

Chapter Six. Bombs

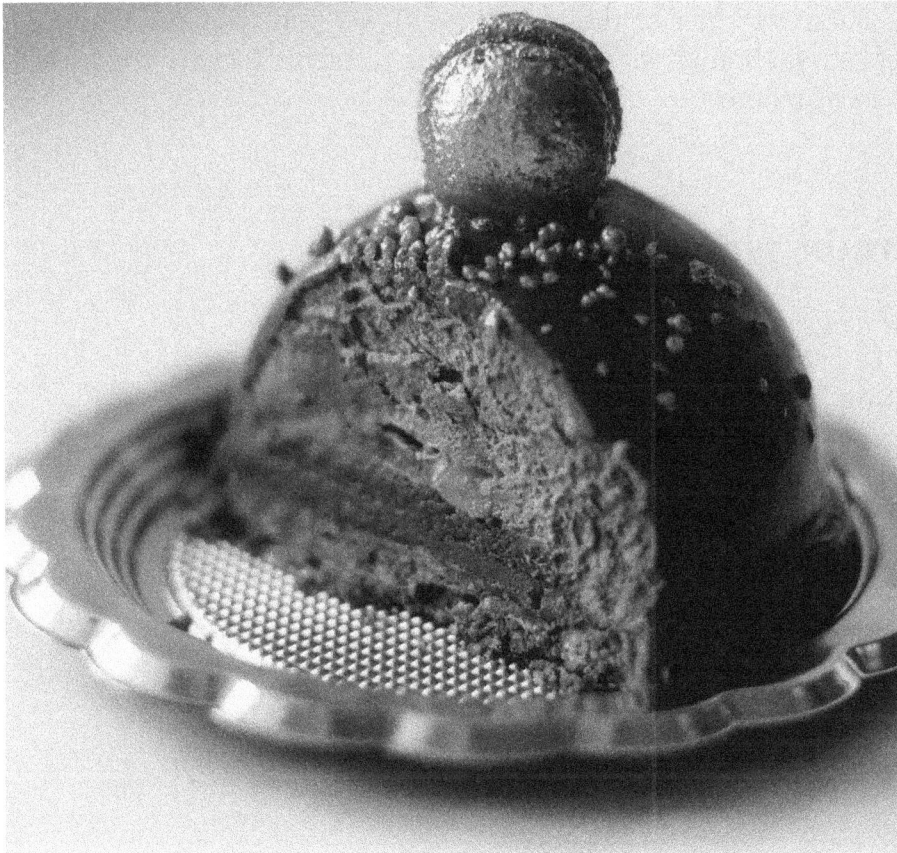

Lemon Almond Chai Fat Bombs

Ingredients

- 65 g coconut oil

- 60 g almond butter, unsweetened and salt-free

- 3 tbsp pistachios, hooked

- 1/2 tbsp swerve sugar substitute

- lemon

- extract almond extract

- Chai spice mixture to taste

Preparations

1. When the coconut oil is solid, heat it slightly until it liquefies. Mix all ingredients except the pistachios. Submerge half of the pistachios. Then pour the mass into silicone molds and garnish the keto fat bombs with the remaining pistachios. Leave the little treats in the fridge for at least half an hour.

Keto Fat Bombs with Cocoa and Chili

Ingredients

- 1 avocado 80g
- coconut
- oil 30g cocoa powder
- 1/2 tsp vanilla extract
- 1 tsp red chilli powder
- 1/2 tsp salt
- 2 tbsp swerve sugar substitute

Preparation

2. When preparing, follow the instructions from the first recipe. Enjoy the healthy fat bombs cooled and garnished as desired with some coarse chili flakes.

Keto Fat Bombs with Tahini and Cocoa

Ingredients

- 8 tbsp pure coconut oil
- 6 tsp sesame seeds, roasted
- 1/4 tsp grape seed
- oil 1/4 tsp sesame oil

- 1/2 tsp salt

- 4 tbsp swerve sugar substitute

- 1 tbsp sesame seeds, black

- 6 tbsp cocoa powder

Preparation

3. For the production of the chocolate layer mix well the coconut oil, the cocoa powder, and the Swerve sugar substitute. Lay out a small mini muffin form with paper cups and fill the hollows up to half with the mass. Allow to cool in the freezer. Except for the sesame, mix the remaining ingredients well. Now pour the Tahini paste over the chocolate base and put the molds back in the freezer. Garnish with black sesame as desired.

Sweet Bomb Keto Almond and Cinnamon

Ingredients:

- ½ cups butter

- ½ cup almond butter (if desired, replace with macadamia butter, tahini, or even coconut fat. See below for almond butter)

- 1 teaspoon vanilla essence

- 1 tablespoon of cinnamon

- Sweetener of your choice (erythritol, stevia, sucralose, whatever you can afford)

Method of Preparation:

1. In a pan, melt butter and almond butter (if you choose erythritol, put it here). Take it off the fire.

2. Add vanilla and cinnamon. Stir well and allow to cool slightly.

3. Add the sweetener (if it is stevia or sucralose).

4. Put in muffin or ice cups.

5. Refrigerate for 30min or 1H.

Tiramisu Fat Bombs

Ingredients

- ¼ cup + 2 tbsp (54g) coconut flour

- ¼ cup (48g) classic monk fruit sweetener, divided

- 1/16 tsp cinnamon

- ½ cup hot water

- ¼ cup (56g) melted butter

- 2 tsp (4g) espresso powder

- 4 oz cream cheese, softened

- ¼ cup (56g) butter, softened

- ¼ cup (64g) No-Sugar-Added SunButter, room temperature

- 1 tbsp pinot noir

- 1 tsp pure vanilla extract

- ¾ tsp (3.75g) cocoa powder

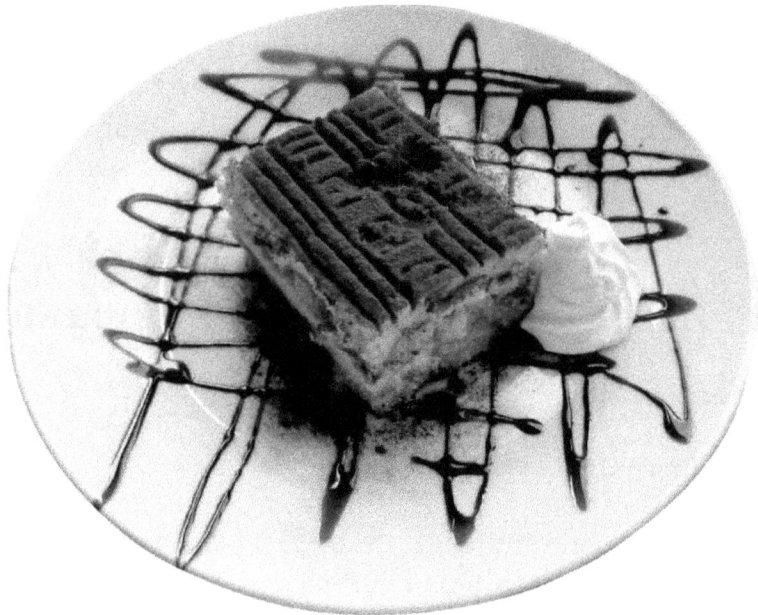

Instructions

1. Put in a small pan over medium heat and toast for about 5 minutes until the coconut flavor becomes golden and fragrant, stir frequently.

2. In a small mixing bowl, mix toasted coconut flour, 1 tablespoon of monk fruit sweetener, and cinnamon. Add hot water, melted butter, espresso, and mix with a fork until well mixed. Spoon the mixture into a silicone mold hole and push it into a flat layer with your fingers. Transfer the silicon mold to a freezer and cool.

3. Meanwhile, add cream cheese, butter, sun butter, and 3 tablespoons of monk fruit sweetener, pino noir, and vanilla extract to the mixing bowl. Using an electric mixer, mix until the ingredients are fully combined. Cover the bowl with a lid or wrap and transfer to the refrigerator for 15 minutes.

4. When the cream cheese mixture has cooled, remove the silicone mold from the freezer and place the cream cheese mixture in the silicone mold above the crust mixture. Sprinkle cocoa

powder on top. Return the silicone mold to the freezer for about 2 hours until the fat bomb becomes solid and can easily jump out of the silicone mold.

Chicken and Pear Salad

Ingredients

- Escarole, canons, or watercress
- Grilled chicken
- Pear
- Pistachios
- sweet onion (rings)
- Pink pepper
- Pink salt
- Extra virgin olive oil 3 tablespoons
- 1 teaspoon Dijon mustard in grain
- 1 teaspoon honey

Instructions

1. Clean and cut delicious escarole or any other green leafy vegetable such as canons, watercress to which you add a few pieces of pear cut into segments or squares.

2. Add chopped pistachios.

3. You can use any other dried fruit that you like more or that you have in the pantry: pine nuts, pecans, almonds.

4. Peel and chop onion, which gives it a spicy point always.

5. And if you dare with the vinaigrette mix, a teaspoon of Dijon mustard in grain, a teaspoon of honey, extra virgin olive oil, lime juice and salt, and pink pepper.

6. Pink pepper is an ingredient that gives an extraordinary touch, in my opinion, and you can crush some and others you leave them whole.

7. The so-called pink pepper, in reality, is the grain of a Brazilian pepper shaker. Its flavor is very peculiar, the mixture of sweet, citrus, little spicy flavor, reminiscent of pine.

8. Finally, you add the roast chicken that you can buy well packed or remains of some homemade preparation.

Salad in Balsamic Tempeh Pot, Strawberries, and Cucumber

Ingredients:

- 240 g. of tempeh nature
- 1/4 cup of tamari
- 1/4 cup of maple syrup
- 1/4 cup of water
- 1/4 cup of balsamic vinegar
- 1 French shallot finely chopped
- 1/3 cup of nutritional yeast
- 1 tbsp. mustard dijon
- 1 tbsp. vegetable oil table
- 1 c. olive oil
- 1/3 cup lemon juice
- 1 cup strawberries diced
- 1 cup English cucumber diced
- 2 cups red lettuce coarsely chopped
- 1/3 cup ground seeds grilled pumpkin
- Salt and pepper

Preparation:

1. In a cauldron filled with boiling water, cook the tempeh for ten minutes. Drain and let stand for 1 to 2 minutes. Cut the boiled tempeh block into cubes and set aside.

2. In a bowl, add tamari, maple syrup, water, balsamic vinegar, French shallot, nutritional yeast, and Dijon mustard. Mix and reserve.

3. In a skillet over medium heat, add the vegetable oil and color the cubes of tempeh. Once lightly browned, pour all the ingredients from your bowl onto the cubes, then bring to a boil by raising the temperature of the pan to medium/high. Mix from time to time until all the liquid has evaporated. Reserve in a bowl.

4. In 2 Mason jars, divide olive oil and lemon juice equitably. Salt and pepper. Assemble the pots in equal portions and steps, adding diced strawberries, English cucumber cubes, tempeh cubes, leaf lettuce leaves, and roasted pumpkin seeds.

5. Store the Mason jars in the fridge and hang them with you in your lunches, in the park, or just for a quick meal on the way home from work. Turn the pot upside down, pour it into a bowl, mix, and enjoy immediately.

Sea Bass and Peppers Salad

Ingredients

- Seabass very clean: A fillet of 150 g.

- Assorted lettuces: 100 g.

- Chives: To taste

- Fresh or roasted red pepper: 1

- Cherry tomatoes to taste

- Garlic clove and parsley 1

- Leek 1

- Carrot 1

- Olive oil One tablespoon

- Salt and lemon to taste

Directions

1. We put the fillet of sea bass in aluminum foil. In the mortar, chop the garlic and parsley, add 2 small teaspoons of oil and cover the fillet of sea bass with it.

2. We also put some leek and carrot strips on the sea bass fillet (the vegetable ribbons can be made with the fruit peeler) and a little salt. Now we close the foil tightly and take it into the oven at 120 ºC for 8-10 minutes. Once cooked, let it cool.

3. In a salad bowl, we put the lettuce mixture and chop the chives and pepper very finely. We add it too. Add the cherry tomatoes cut into quarters. Add only a small teaspoon of olive oil, salt, and lemon as a dressing, and now add the fish with the vegetables we have cooked in the oven and ready to eat.

Thai Beef Salad Tears of the Tiger

Ingredients

- 800 g of beef tenderloin

- For the marinade:

- 2 tablespoons of soy sauce

- 1 tablespoon soup of honey

- 1 pinch of the pepper mill

- For the sauce:

- 1 small bunch of fresh coriander

- 1 small bouquet of mint

- 3 tablespoons soup of fish sauce

- lemon green

- 1 clove of garlic

- tablespoons soup of sugar palm (or brown sugar)

- 1 bird pepper or ten drops of Tabasco

- 1 small glass of raw Thai rice to make grilled rice powder

- 200 g of arugula or young shoots of salad

Preparation

1. Cut the beef tenderloin into strips and put it in a container. Sprinkle with 2 tablespoons soy sauce, 1 tablespoon honey, and pepper. Although soak thoroughly and let marinate 1 hour at room temperature.

2. Meanwhile, prepare the roasted rice powder. Pour a glass of Thai rice into an anti-adhesive pan. Dry color the rice, constantly stirring to avoid burning. When it has a lovely color, get rid of it on a plate and let it cool.

3. When it has cooled, reduce it to powder by mixing it with the robot.

4. Wash and finely chop mint and coriander. Put in a container and add lime juice, chopped garlic clove, 3 tablespoons Nuoc mam, 3 tablespoons brown sugar, 3 tablespoons water, 1 tablespoon sauce soy, and a dozen drops of Tabasco. Mix well and let stand the time that the sugar melts and the flavors mix.

5. Place a bed of salad on a dish. Cook the beef strips put them on the salad. Sprinkle with the spoonful of sauce and roasted rice powder. To be served as is or with a Thai cooked white rice scented.

Coconut Shakshuka

Preparation: 20 min

Ready in 45 min

Ingredients

- 80 g large onions (1 large onion)

- 3 garlic cloves

- 2 red peppers

- 10 g coriander (0.5 bunch)

- 3 tbsp olive oil

- 600 g chunky tomatoes (can)

- 70 g desiccated coconut (8 tbsp)

- 60 ml coconut milk (4 tbsp)

- salt

- pepper

- 1 tsp ground cumin

- 1 tsp sweet paprika powder

- 2 tsp curry powder

- piri-piri (chili spice)

- 4 eggs

Preparation steps

1. Peel onion and garlic and chop finely. Halve, core, wash, and dice the peppers. Wash the coriander, shake dry and remove the leaves.

2. Heat the oil in a large pan. Sauté onion and pepper cubes in it, stirring, for about 10 minutes over medium heat. Then stir in the garlic, tomatoes, desiccated coconut, and coconut milk. Season the sauce with salt, pepper, cumin, paprika powder, curry powder, and about ¼ teaspoon piri piri to taste and simmer for 20 minutes over low heat until thick.

3. Beat the eggs one after the other, slide into the sauce and cover and let set for about 5 minutes over low heat. Sprinkle the tomato and egg pan with piri piri and coriander and serve.

Fish Curry with Coconut Milk and Rice

Preparation: 30 min

Ready in 50 min

Ingredients

- 1 onion

- 10 g ginger (1 piece)

- 3 tomatoes

- 600 g white fish fillet (ready to cook, skinless; e.g. monkfish, cod)

- 3 tbsp lime juice

- 1 pinch ground coriander

- 300 g basmati rice

- 2 tbsp germ oil

- 1 tbsp red curry paste

- 400 ml of coconut milk

- salt

- pepper

- 1 tbsp fish sauce

- 2 stems coriander

Preparation steps

1. Cut the onion and ginger finely and peel. Cut the tomatoes and cut into small cubes, wash, quarter and core. Wash the fish as well, toss dry and cut into large pieces in bite-size. Mix the lime juice and the coriander, drizzle the fillet, allow to steep for approximately 30 minutes. Cook the rice in the meantime following packet instructions.

2. Heat the oil in a pan, let the fish pieces drain a bit (collect marinade, set aside) and fry in the hot oil until golden and then remove them.

3. Steam onion in the roasting fat, sauté briefly and pour into the cocoon's milk, stir into the curry paste. Gently cook about 10 minutes over medium heat, then add the fish and tomatoes and cook for 2-3 more minutes. Finally, add salt, pepper, and fish to the lime marinade.

4. On 4 preheated plates, arrange the rice curry. Wash coriander, dry, pluck, and add curry. Wash coriander, shake dry. Serve straight away.

Chapter Seven Cakes

Blueberry and Banana Muffins

Preparation: 25 min Ready in 1 h

ingredients

- 1 small organic lemon

- 200 g wheat flour type 1050

- 5 tbsp wheat bran

- 2 tsp baking powder

- 80 g coconut blossom sugar

- 1 pinch salt

- 150 ml milk (1.5% fat)

- 1 egg

- 2 tbsp rapeseed oil

- 250 g ripe small bananas (2 ripe small bananas)

- 175 g blueberries

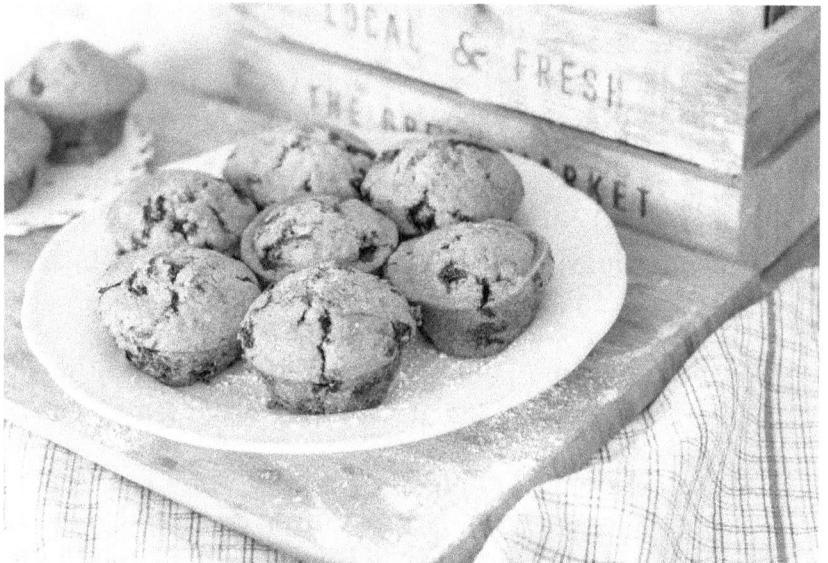

Preparation steps

1. Rinse the lemon and rub the peel in the hot water. In a bowl, place the flour, bran, bakery pulse, cocoon flowers and a little bit of salt. Thoroughly mix it all.

2. Beat milk, egg, and oil in a second bowl until they are smooth. Add the meal blend and mix into a smooth dough.

3. Peel and smooth the bananas with a bifurcation. Fill in the batter with the banana puree and thoroughly mix.

4. Add the batter, sort and fold in the blueberries.

5. Line a covered muffin tin with a bakery of paper (for twelve muffins). Disseminate the batter in the molds.

6. Bake the muffins in a pre-heated oven for about 30 minutes at a temperature of 200 ° C (fan oven: 180 ° C, gas level 3). Take a stick of wooden into the middle of the muffin: if clean, the muffins are ready; bake for a few minutes otherwise.

7. With the paper liners, remove the muffins from the tin. Cool down on a wire rack, and serve tidy or cold for at least 5 minutes.

Marbled Strawberry Cake with Amaretto

Preparation: 1 h

ready in 16 h 30 min

ingredients

- 650 g yogurt (1.5% fat)

- 3 eggs

- 1 pinch salt

- 90 g coconut blossom sugar

- 60 g flour (type 1050)

- 1 pinch baking powder

- 3 tbsp ground almond kernels

- 1 small organic orange

- 750 g strawberries

- 12 sheets white gelatin

- 20 g amaretto

- 100 g whipped cream

- 1 tbsp red currant jelly or other red fruit jelly

- 1 packet red cake topping

- 125 ml cherry juice

Preparation steps

1. Into a coffee filter or towel, pour in the yogurt, and let drain overnight in the fridge.

2. Line the bottom with bakery paper of a springform pot (26 cm). Divide the eggs. Beat the egg whites and salt in a high container with a hand mixer's whisk until steep.

3. In a bowl, place the egg yolks and the cocoon flower sucre in 3 tablespoons of warm water. Beat with the mixer's whisk until creamy and thick.

4. In a small bowl, mix the flour and bakery powder and sprinkle with the almonds onto the custard.

5. Add the egg whites to the flour and almond blend and fold into the blanket carefully.

6. In the prepared pan, pour the batter and smooth out somewhat. Bake in the middle rack for 25–30 minutes until golden brown on the pre-heated ovens at 180 ° C (fan oven: 160 ° C, gas: level 2–3).

7. Remove the sponge cake from the mold, and allow the wire rack to fully cool down. In the meantime, rub dry and finely grate 2 teaspoons of the peel, then wash the orange with warm water. Cut the orange half-half and squeeze.

8. In a bowl of water, clean up and dry up kitchen paper carefully, wash the strawberries. On a plate to garnish, chill about 1/4.

9. In a large container, put the remaining berries and puree roughly with the mixer. Sprinkle the gelatine 5 to 7 minutes in cold water.

10. Remove the yogurt in a bowl with the orange peel and four cubs of orange juice.

11. Squeeze the gelatine out and heat until it is dissolved in a small saucepan.

12. Mix the gelatine with 4 tablespoons of the mixture and mix into the rest of the yogurt. Mix it. Mix the amarettini and the mashed strawberries one by one.

13. Pour the cream into a large bowl and beat until stiff with the hand mixer. Fold the yogurt mix loosely to create a pattern like marble.

14. In the microwave or a small cup, heat the currant jelly briefly. Brush the cake with it in a cooled sponge. Sit around the base and close up the springform ring.

15. Put on the dough and smooth the strawberry yoghurt mix. Let the cake harden for approximately 3 hours inside the refrigerator.

16. Following the package instructions, prepare the icing with cherry juice.

17. Add the rest of the strawberries to the cake and decorate with the icing. Serve the cake and let the icing set.

Carrot and Almond Muffins

Preparation: 15 minutes

Ready in 1 h 20 min

Ingredients

- 2 eggs

- 80 g cane sugar

- 80 ml rapeseed oil

- 125 ml buttermilk

- 130 g small carrots (2 small carrots)

- 100 g small apples (1 small apple)

- ½ lemon

- 200 g whole wheat flour

- 70 g ground almond kernels

- 3 tsp tartar baking powder

Preparation steps

1. Put the eggs and sugar in a bowl. Beat with the whisk of a hand mixer until frothy. Stir in the oil and buttermilk.

2. Wash, clean, peel the carrots and grate finely in a bowl on a box grater.

3. Peel, quarter, core, and grate the apple. Squeeze the lemon and mix 1 tbsp lemon juice into the grated apple.

4. Mix the flour, almonds, and baking powder in a bowl. Stir quickly into the egg and sugar mixture. Fold in the carrot and apple rasp with a whisk.

5. Line the 12 hollows of a muffin tin with paper liners and fill in the batter. Bake in the oven at 180 ° C (fan oven 160 ° C, gas: level 2-3) until golden brown for 20-25 minutes.

6. Remove the muffins from the mould with the paper liners. Let cool on a wire rack for 40-60 minutes and serve.

Plum Crispy Cake with Chocolate Base

Preparation: 35 min

Ready in 4 h 35 min

Ingredients

- 80 g dark chocolate (at least 70% cocoa content)

- 50 g cornflakes (unsweetened)

- 8 sheets red gelatin

- 500 g plums

- 1 branch rosemary

- 60 g liquid honey (4 tbsp)

- 200 ml red grape juice

- 250 g low-fat quark

- 100g yoghurt (1.5% fat)

Preparation steps

1. Roughly chop the chocolate, place in a bowl, and melt in a warm water bath or the microwave.

2. Roughly crumble the cornflakes, add to the melted chocolate and stir until all the cornflakes are coated with chocolate.

3. Line the bottom of a small springform pan (18 cm) with baking paper and add the cornflakes. Spread evenly in it and let cool until the chocolate is completely solid.

4. In the meantime, soak the gelatine in cold water.

5. Wash the plums, cut in half, stone and cut into small pieces. Wash rosemary and shake dry.

6. Bring the plums to the boil with rosemary, honey, and grape juice in a saucepan. Reduce the heat and cook over low heat until the plums are soft. Let cool a little and remove the rosemary.

7. Squeeze out the gelatine well, add it to the still warm plums and dissolve while stirring. Coarsely puree with a hand blender and allow to cool completely.

8. Mix the quark and yoghurt with the whisk of a hand mixer until creamy and mix with 2/3 of the plum puree.

9. First, put the plum and quark cream, then the rest of the fruit puree on the base and smooth out each time.

10. Make a marble pattern with a fork and refrigerate the cake for about 4 hours.

Berry Meringue Cake

Preparation: 25 min

Ready in 1 h

Ingredients

- 100 g red currants

- 100 g gooseberries

- 1 tsp food starch

- 150 g flour

- 40 g coconut blossom sugar (2 tbsp)

- ½ tsp ground cardamom

- 1 tsp baking powder

- salt

- 75 ml milk (1.5% fat)

- 2 tbsp rapeseed oil

- 3 eggs (s)

- 1 egg white (s)

- 25 g icing sugar made from erythritol

Preparation steps

1. Wash berries, drain well, clean, and mix in a bowl with starch.

2. Mix the flour, coconut blossom sugar, cardamom, baking powder, and a pinch of salt in a second bowl.

3. In another bowl, whisk together the milk, oil, and 3 eggs with the hand mixer. Add to the flour and stir in briefly.

4. Line the bottom of a small springform pan (18 cm Ø) with baking paper and spread the batter into it.

5. Spread the berries on top and bake in the preheated oven at 180 ° C (convection: 160 ° C, gas: level 2–3) on the middle rack for about 25 minutes.

6. Beat the egg whites with the whisk of the hand mixer to very stiff snow, gradually pour in the erythritol and keep beating for at least 10 minutes (there should be no more erythritol crystals).

7. Spread the egg whites on the cake and bake for another 8–10 minutes. Remove from the mould and let cool down on a wire rack.

Quince Cake

Preparation: 1 h 15 min

Ingredients

- 4 eggs

- 1 pinch salt

- 60 g raw cane sugar (4 tbsp)

- 50 g whole wheat flour

- 50 g food starch

- 15 g cocoa powder (1 tbsp)

- 800 g quinces

- 1 vanilla pod

- ½ lemon

- 150 ml apple syrup

- 200 ml apple juice

- 2 packages clear cake topping

- 2 sheets white gelatin

- 300 g low-fat quark

- 200 g yoghurt (3.5% fat)

- cinnamon (to taste)

Preparation steps

1. Separate eggs. Put the egg white, salt, and 2 tablespoons of raw cane sugar in a tall container. Beat with the whisk of the hand mixer to a stiff snow.

2. Beat the egg yolks with the remaining raw cane sugar and 3 tablespoons of hot water in a bowl for about 4 minutes until thick and creamy.

3. Put the flour, starch, and cocoa in a fine sieve and sift into a second bowl. Fold alternately with egg whites under the egg yolk cream.

4. Line the bottom and edge of a springform pan (24 cm) with baking paper. Pour in the sponge cake and smooth it out. Bake in a preheated oven at 200 ° C (convection 180 ° C; gas: level 3) for about 8-10 minutes.

5. Let cool on a wire rack. Detach the bottom from the mould and put the edge around it again.

6. Wash the quinces and peel them with a peeler. Quarter with a large knife, remove the core, cut into thin slices, and place in a saucepan.

7. Halve the vanilla pod lengthways and scrape out the pulp. Squeeze the lemon and measure 2 tablespoons of juice.

8. Add the vanilla pulp and lemon juice with apple syrup and apple juice to the quince. Bring to the boil and cook over a low heat for about 10 minutes.

9. Drain the quinces well in a sieve (catching the juice) and place on the cake base.

10. Prepare the icing according to the instructions on the packet with cooking liquid and water. Pour over quince and chill.

11. Soak the gelatine in cold water. Stir the quark with yoghurt until smooth and add cinnamon to taste.

12. Heat dripping wet gelatine in a small saucepan and dissolve while stirring.

13. Stir about 1/3 of the quark mass into the warm gelatin and then immediately stir into the rest of the mixture.

14. Spread the mixture on the quince and chill the cake for at least 2 hours.

15. To serve, loosen the rim and place the quince cake on a plate. If you like, put the cinnamon in a tea strainer and dust over it.

Fruit Curd Cake

Preparation: 40 min

Ready in 2 h

Ingredients

- 230 g flour

- 5 g dry yeast (1 packet)

- 200 ml milk (1.5% fat)

- 60 g sugar (3 tbsp)

- 250 g bright grapes

- 250 g elderberries

- 15 g butter (1 tbsp)

- 4 eggs (size m)

- 150 g sour cream

- 150 g low-fat quark

- 1 packet vanilla sugar

Preparation steps

1. Mix the flour and yeast thoroughly in a bowl. Warm milk and add lukewarm with 2 teaspoons of sugar. Knead into a smooth dough with the dough hook of the hand mixer.

2. Cover and let rise in a warm place for 30-40 minutes, until the batter has about doubled.

3. In the meantime, wash the grapes and elderberries, drain them well and pluck them from the stems.

4. Briefly knead the dough again with your hands. Roll out into a circle (approx. 32 cm) on a floured work surface.

5. Grease a tart or pizza pan (30 cm) with the butter. Place the dough in the mould, pull up one edge all around and press down a little.

6. Spread the fruit on the dough. Whisk the eggs, sour cream, quark, remaining sugar, and vanilla sugar in a second bowl with the whisk of the hand mixer and pour-over.

7. Bake the cake in the preheated oven at 180 ° C (fan oven: 160 ° C; gas: level 2-3) on the lowest rack for 40-45 minutes. Let cool in the tin on a wire rack.

Warm Apple Cake

Preparation: 30 min

Ready in 1 h 20 min

Ingredients

- 100 g butter

- 80 g coconut blossom sugar

- ½ tsp vanilla powder

- 1 pinch salt

- 3 eggs (size m)

- ½ organic lemon

- 2 tbsp maple syrup

- 200 g whole wheat flour

- 1 tsp baking powder

- ½ tsp cinnamon powder

- 50 g applesauce

- 3 tbsp milk (3.5% fat)

- 800 g apples

- 2 tbsp sunflower seeds

Preparation steps

1. Beat soft butter with coconut blossom sugar until frothy, add vanilla powder, and salt. Stir eggs one after the other into the mixture. Wash the lemon with hot water, pat dry, rub off the peel and squeeze out the juice. Add lemon zest to the butter mixture and stir in.

2. Mix the flour with baking powder and cinnamon and stir alternately with the applesauce and milk into the butter mixture in portions until a smooth dough is formed. Peel, halve, core the apples, and cut thinly into the surface. Mix the apple halves with the lemon juice and maple syrup.

3. Pour the batter into a springform pan that has been greased if necessary, smooth it out, and place the apple halves on the batter with the smooth sides facing down. Scatter sunflower seeds over the top and bake in a preheated oven at 180 ° C (fan oven: 160 ° C; gas: level 2–3) for about 50 minutes.

Chocolate Cupcake with Almonds

Preparation: 10 min

Ingredients

- 75 g wheat flour type 1050

- 1 tbsp almonds (roasted and ground)

- 15 g cocoa powder

- 25 g raw cane sugar

- ¼ tsp baking powder

- 2 pinches ground tonka bean

- 25 g butter

- 6 tbsp milk (3.5% fat)

- 2 tsp chocolate drops (dark)

- 1 tsp almonds

Preparation steps

1. Put the flour, almonds, cocoa, sugar, baking powder, and tonka bean in a small bowl and stir carefully.

2. Melt butter in the microwave at 600 watts for 1 minute. Stir liquid butter, milk, and chocolate chips into the flour mixture. Pour the dough into two small cups and smooth out a little.

3. Place the mug cake in the microwave for 1 minute and 30 seconds at 800 watts. If the cupcakes are still too soft, put them in for another 30 seconds. Finely chop the almonds, sprinkle with the cupcake and enjoy warm.

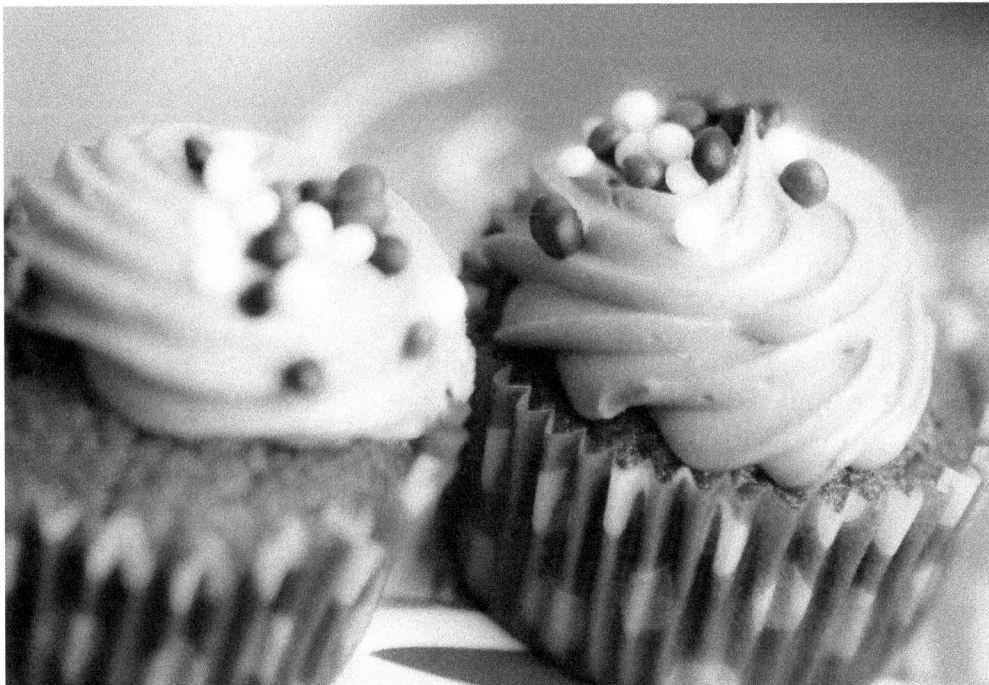

Hazelnut Cake

Preparation: 25 min

Ready in 1 h 5 min

Ingredients

- 1 apple

- 150 g ground hazelnuts

- 1 ½ tsp baking powder

- 100 g spelled flour type 1050

- ½ organic orange

- 3 eggs

- 1 ½ tsp honey

- 100 g butter

- 100 g applesauce (no added sugar)

- 75 g almond kernels

- 1 tbsp almond flakes

Preparation steps

1. Wash the apple and grate it finely. Mix hazelnuts with baking powder and spelled flour, then fold into the apples. Wash the orange with hot water, rub dry, rub the peel and squeeze out the juice.

2. Separate eggs. Beat egg whites very stiff. Beat the egg yolks with 1 tbsp orange juice, honey, and butter until frothy. Stir into the apple-nut mixture together with the orange peel and applesauce. Roughly chop the almonds and carefully fold into the dough with the egg whites.

3. Place the dough in a spring form lined with baking paper and bake at 180 ° C (convection 160 ° C; gas: level 2-3) for about 40 minutes. Carry out a stick test, take the cake out of the oven and let it cool in the pan.

Pineapple and Carrot Cake

Preparation: 40 min

Ready in 1 h 10 min

Ingredients

- 300 g fresh pineapple (1 piece)

- 200 g carrots (2 carrots)

- 4 eggs

- 80 g sugar

- 150 g ground almond kernels

- 80 g flour

- 1 tsp baking powder

- ½ tsp cinnamon

- 50 g walnut kernels

- 50 g plum jam (with sweetener)

- 1 tbsp powdered sugar

Preparation steps

1. Peel and dice the pineapple. Wash, peel, and grate the carrots on a grater.

2. Separate the eggs. Put the egg whites in a bowl or a tall vessel and beat until stiff with the whisk of the hand mixer, gradually pouring in 40 g of sugar.

3. Whip the egg yolks with the rest of the sugar in a bowl until creamy.

4. Mix the almonds, flour, baking powder, and cinnamon in a bowl.

5. Use a whisk to fold the flour mixture and egg whites into the egg yolk mixture.

6. Chop walnuts with a large knife. Mix with the carrots, pineapple, and plum jam and fold into the batter with a wooden spoon.

7. Line a baking sheet with parchment paper and spread the dough on it with a palette. Bake in the preheated oven at 180 ° C (convection: 160 °, gas: level 2-3) on the middle rack for 20-25 minutes.

8. Put the powdered sugar in a tea strainer, dust the warm cake with it and let it cool on an oven rack. Cut into pieces and serve.

Lactose-free Cheesecake

Ingredients

- 180 g whole wheat biscuit (or oatmeal biscuit)

- 110 g coconut oil

- 45 g hearty oat flakes

- 750 g lactose-free skimmed quark

- 1 organic lemon

- 1 vanilla pod

- 200 g lactose-free cream cheese (double cream level; at least 60% fat in dry matter)

- 90 g coconut blossom sugar

- 4 eggs (size m)

- 40 g food starch

Preparation steps

1. In a clean tea towel, place the biscuits and use the rolling pine for crumbling. In a small cup of coconut oil, mix with the chips and oatmeal over a low heating.

2. Line the baked paper in the springform breadcrumbs. Pour the mixture into the biscuit and squeeze it down.

3. Drain quark well. Drain quark well. Rinse the lemon with hot water, toss it dry and rub the peel thoroughly. Cut the lemon half and the juice out. Split the vanilla pod and scrape the pulp out.

4. To top it, add quark, lemon peel and juice, vanilla pulp, cream cheese, and cocoa flower sugar. Remove the eggs one by one. Use starch briefly.

5. On the base of the cookie, put the topping. In a pre-heated oven, cook for 50-60 minutes at 180 ° C (convection 160 ° C; gas: 2-3) Take it out and let it cool. Serve in pieces. Serve.

Beetroot and Cocoa Cake

Preparation: 50 min

Ingredients

- 300 g beetroot (2 bulbs)
- 1 apple
- 3 eggs
- 50 g maple syrup
- 1 pinch salt
- cinnamon
- 110 g soft butter
- 125 g wholemeal spelled flour
- 125 g spelled flour type 630
- 1 tsp baking powder
- 30 g heavily de-oiled cocoa powder (3 tbsp)
- 100 ml milk (3.5% fat)
- 50 g dark chocolate (at least 70% cocoa content)
- 30 g hazelnut kernels (2 tbsp)

Preparation steps

1. Peel and finely grate the beetroot tubers. Clean, wash, quarter, core, and roughly grate the apple.

2. Beat the eggs with maple syrup, a pinch of salt, and 1/4 teaspoon cinnamon until frothy. Add 100 g butter and continue beating.

3. Mix both types of flour with baking powder and cocoa powder, add to the egg mixture and stir. Add milk and work everything into a smooth dough. Fold the beetroot and grated apple into the batter.

4. Grease a springform pan with the remaining butter. Pour in the dough, smooth it out and bake in a preheated oven at 200 ° C (fan oven 180 ° C; gas: level 3) for 35–40 minutes. Take out of the oven and let cool for 15 minutes.

Quick Coconut Cake

Preparation: 30 min

Ready in 45 min

Ingredients

- 200 g flour

- 200 g sugar

- ½ packet baking powder

- 250 ml buttermilk

- 2 eggs

- 50 g desiccated coconut

- 300 g small ripe mango (1 small ripe mango)

- 100 g yoghurt (1.5% fat)

- 2 passion fruit

Preparation steps

1. Mix the flour, 150 g sugar, and baking powder in a bowl.

2. Thoroughly whisk the buttermilk and eggs together and stir into the flour mixture.

3. Line a square baking pan (24x24 cm) with baking paper. Pour in the dough and smooth it out with a rubber spatula.

4. Mix the coconut flakes and the remaining sugar in a small bowl and sprinkle over the dough. Bake in the preheated oven at 180 ° C (convection: 160 ° C, gas: level 2-3) on the middle shelf for 20-25 minutes.

5. In the meantime, peel the mango, cut the pulp off the stone in slices, dice, and stir with the yoghurt until smooth.

6. Halve the passion fruit and scoop out with a teaspoon. Add the pulp to the yoghurt and serve with the warm cake.

Apple Brownies with Vanilla

Preparation: 15 minutes

Ready in 40 min

Ingredients

- 2 eggs

- 1 pinch salt

- 60 g coconut blossom sugar

- 1 vanilla pod

- 175 g applesauce (without sugar)

- 100 g spelled flour type 1050

- ½ tsp baking powder

- 20 g cocoa powder (1 heaped tablespoon)

- 1 tsp icing sugar made from birch sugar (as desired)

Preparation steps

1. Separate the eggs. Put the egg whites in a tall container, egg yolks in a bowl. Add a little salt to the egg white and use the hand mixer to beat until stiff, gradually pouring in the coconut blossom sugar.

2. Halve the vanilla pod lengthways with a small, pointed knife and scrape out the pulp.

3. Stir the vanilla pulp and applesauce into the egg yolks with a wooden spoon.

4. Mix the flour, baking powder, and cocoa powder in a bowl and sift into the egg yolk mixture. Mix in briefly, then fold in the egg whites.

5. Line the bottom of a square baking pan (20x20 cm) with parchment paper. Pour in the dough and smooth it out with a rubber spatula.

6. Bake in a preheated oven at 175 ° C (fan oven: 150 ° C, gas: level 2) for about 20 minutes. Pierce the middle of the dough with a wooden skewer: if it comes out clean, the dough is done; otherwise bake for a few minutes.

7. Remove the mold and let the brownies cool for 5 minutes. Then remove the dough from the mold and let cool down completely on a wire rack.

8. Using a large knife, cut into 9 equal squares. Put powdered sugar in a tea strainer and dust the brownies with it.

Chapter Eight. Pies and Tarts

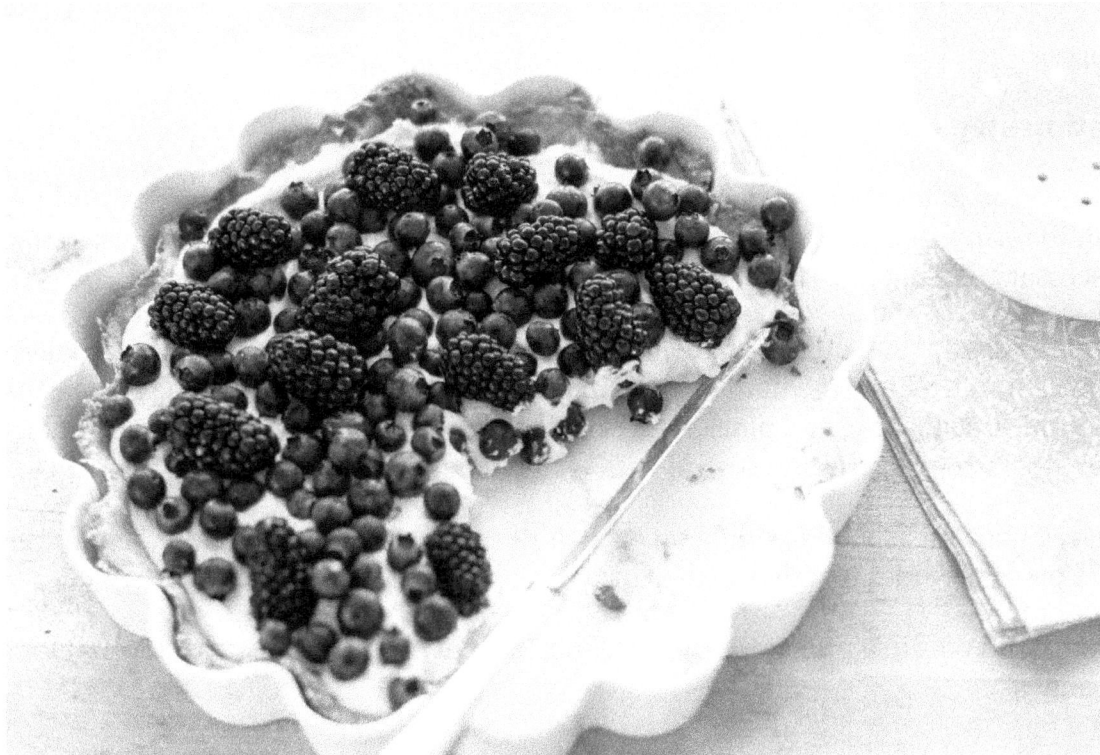

Hand Pies with a Tomato

Preparation: 40 min

Ready in 1 h

Ingredients

- 200 g wholemeal spelled flour + 2 tbsp for processing

- 150 g vegetable yogurt alternative made from soy

- 3 tsp olive oil

- 2 tsp baking powder

- salt

- 1 shallot

- 90 g tomato paste (6 tbsp)

- 2 branches rosemary

- 45 g hazelnut kernels (3 tbsp)

- pepper

Preparation steps

1. Knead 200 g flour with yogurt alternative, 2 teaspoons oil, baking powder, and 1 pinch of salt to form a dough. Roll out the dough about ½ cm thin on a floured work surface if necessary and cut out 12 circles with a diameter of about 8 cm with a glass.

2. Peel the shallot and dice very finely. Heat the remaining oil in a pan. Sauté shallot cubes in it for 2 minutes over medium heat. Remove from heat and mix with tomato paste. Wash rosemary, shake dry, and pluck needles. Finely chop the rosemary and hazelnuts, add to the tomato paste mixture, and season with salt and pepper.

3. Place about 1 teaspoon of filling on each of the dough circles, then fold them in the middle and press the sides together with a fork.

4. Bake hand pies in a preheated oven at 200 ° C (fan oven: 180 ° C; gas: level 3) for 20 minutes.

Pecan Pie Cheesecake in a Glass

Preparation: 40 min

Ingredients

- 100 g whole grain biscuit

- 100 g pecans

- 40 g liquid butter

- ½ tsp cinnamon powder

- 1 vanilla pod

- 300 g cream cheese

- 300 g low-fat quark

- 2 eggs

- 3 tbsp honey

- 1 tbsp food starch

- 2 tbsp raw cane sugar

- 50 ml whipped cream

- coarse sea salt as required

Preparation steps

1. In a clean tea towel, place the biscuits and use the rolling pine for crumbing. Cut approximately 25 grams of nuts finely and mix in butter, crumbs, and cinnamon. Into the glasses and press the biscuit mixture firmly.

2. Halve the vanilla pod longitudinally and smash out with a knife the vanilla pulp. Put in a hand blender, mix the vanilla pulp, cream cheese, fatty quark, eggs, sweet mixture, and cornstarch.

3. Spread on the glasses the cheese mix. Place the glasses in a high baker and fill the pot of hot water to allow the water to reach the middle of the glasses. Cook the cheese in a preheated oven for about thirty minutes, at 180 ° C (fan oven 160 ° C; gas level 2–3). Take it out and let it cool.

4. Cut the remainder of the nuts grossly. In the saucepan put raw cane sugar, heat, and caramelize over medium heat. Add the cream, stir, and add 1-2 minutes. Remove. Fill the rest of the nuts.

5. Decorate a dollop of nut caramel with cheesecake and, if necessary, cover it with coarse sea salt.

Whoopie Pies with Blueberries

Preparation: 30 min, ready in 45 min

Ingredients

For the dough

- 125 g butter

- 100 g sugar

- 2 eggs

- 1 pinch lemon peel

- 250 g flour

- 1 tsp vanilla pudding powder

- 1 tsp baking powder

- 125 g blueberries

For the cream

- 200 g whipped cream at least 30% fat

- 1 packet cream stiffener

- 1 tbsp powdered sugar

Preparation steps

1. Top and bottom heat preheat the oven to 180 ° C. Mix together the butter and stir into sugar, eggs, and lemon zest all the time. Stir in the mix. Mix the flour and pudding powder, mix and mix. Fold the blueberries carefully. Place the mixture in a pipe bag on a baking sheet, fasten with a large punch and squirt 2-3 cm blobs with sufficient space between them. Bake for 10-15 minutes in the preheated oven. Remove the paper from the plate, remove it, and leave the pieces on a wire rack cool.
Whip the cream to semi-rigid for the cream. In the cream, add the cream stiffener and the powdered sugar and whip. Keep beating until the cream is rugged. Brush with cream half the pieces and put a suitable lid on top. Click and serve lightly.

Potato Tart

Preparation: 40 min

Ingredients

- 1 kg waxy potatoes

- salt

- 300 g whole wheat flour

- 5 eggs

- 2 tbsp vegetable oil

- 300 ml whipped cream

- 3 tbsp creme fraiche cheese

- pepper

- nutmeg

- 20 g liquid butter

Preparation steps

1. Wash the potatoes and pre-cook them in salted boiling water for 15 minutes. In the meantime, mix 280 g of flour with salt, sieve on a work surface, make a well in the middle, pour in 1 egg, oil, and 125 ml of lukewarm water, and quickly work all the ingredients into a smooth dough with your hands. If necessary, add a little more water or flour. Shape into a ball and let rest under a heated bowl for 30 minutes.

2. Mix the cream with the remaining eggs and crème fraîche and season with salt, pepper, and nutmeg. Drain the potatoes, rinse, peel, and let cool completely.

3. Spread out a kitchen towel and sprinkle with the remaining flour, put the dough on top, roll out a little, and then pull out as thin as possible over the back of your hand. Cut off the thick edges of the dough. Grease the tart pan if necessary and place the batter in it. Fold the protruding dough outwards.

4. Cut the potatoes into thin slices and mix carefully with the egg cream. Spread on the strudel dough and fold in the protruding dough pieces in the middle so that the potato mixture is completely covered. Spread smoothly, brush with liquid butter and bake in a preheated oven at 180 ° C (fan oven 160 ° C; gas: level 2–3) for 35–40 minutes until golden brown. Take out, let cool down briefly, carefully remove from the mold, and serve cut into pieces.

Whoopie Pies with Chocolate Cream

Preparation: 30 min

Ready in 45 min

Ingredients

For the dough

- 125 g butter

- 100 g sugar

- 2 eggs

- 1 pinch lemon peel

- 250 g flour

- 1 tsp vanilla pudding powder

- 1 tsp baking powder

For the cream

- 100 g dark couverture

- 30 g butter in flakes

- 2 tbsp whipped cream at least 30% fat content

Preparation steps

1. Preheat the oven to 180 ° C top and bottom heat. Mix the butter until white and creamy and gradually stir in the sugar, eggs, and lemon zest. Mix the flour with the baking powder and the pudding powder and stir in as well.

2. Pour the mixture into a piping bag and squirt small blobs (approx. 2 cm in diameter) with enough space between them on a baking sheet lined with baking paper. Bake in the preheated oven for 10-15 minutes. Remove, remove the baking paper from the tray, and let the cakes cool on a wire rack.

3. For the cream, melt the chocolate over a hot, non-boiling water bath, remove from the water bath and let cool slightly. Stir in the butter and cream and let the mixture cool down. Brush half of the whoopie pies with the cream and place a suitable counterpart on top. Press lightly and serve.

Chocolate Whoopies

Preparation: 1 h

Ready in 1 h 25 min

Ingredients

For the dough

- 125 g flour

- 35 g food starch

- 35 g cocoa powder

- 1 tsp baking powder

- 100 g soft butter

- 80 g powdered sugar

- 1 tsp vanilla sugar

- 1 egg

- 100 ml buttermilk

For the filling

- 1 protein

- 1 pinch salt

- ½ tsp baking powder

- 80 g sugar

Preparation steps

1. Preheat the oven to 160 ° C fan oven. Line two baking trays with parchment paper. Mix the flour with the starch, cocoa, and baking powder. Whisk the butter until creamy and sift the powdered sugar. Add the vanilla sugar and whisk in. Mix in the egg and buttermilk thoroughly. Sift the flour mixture and stir in. Fill into a piping bag with a round nozzle and spray about 30 circles on the baking sheets with a little space between them. Bake in the oven for about 15 minutes. Then remove and let cool on a wire rack.

2. For the cream, beat the egg white, salt, and baking powder for at least 5 minutes until stiff. Bring the sugar to the boil with 80 ml of water in a saucepan over high heat while stirring and let it boil down for about 10 minutes until thick. Continue to stir the egg white on the lowest level of the mixer and slowly pour in the hot sugar syrup. Stir the cream for another 5 minutes. Then fill a piping bag with a perforated nozzle and spray on 15 whoopie bottoms. Cover with the rest of the whoopies. If desired, lightly flame the edges with a bunsen burner and serve.

Cream Cheese and Berry Tart

Preparation: 40 min

Ingredients

- 1 organic lemon

- 200 g zwieback

- 100 yoghurt butter (room temperature)

- 6 sheets white gelatin

- 50 g sugar

- 600 g cream cheese preparation (0.2% fat)

- 2 protein

- 400 g mixed berries (e.g. blueberries, blackberries, currants)

Preparation steps

1. Line a springform pan (26 cm) with cling film.

2. Wash lemon with hot water, pat dry, rub off 1 pinch of peel, squeeze out the juice.

3. Crumble the rusk and mix well with the butter and lemon zest. Press evenly on the bottom of the pan and place in the refrigerator.

4. soak the gelatine in cold water. Mix 4 tablespoons of lemon juice with sugar and cream cheese until smooth.

5. Dissolve the gelatine dripping wet in a saucepan over low heat. Mix first with 3 tablespoons of cream cheese, then with the rest of the cream cheese.

6. Separate eggs (use egg yolks otherwise). Beat the egg whites until stiff, fold into the cream cheese cream, spread on the rusk base, and smooth out. Chill for at least 3 hours.

7. In the meantime, wash the berries and drain them well. Detach the tart from the mold, remove the foil. Spread the berries on the tart.

Zucchini Chorizo Cheese Tart

Ingredient

For the dough:

- 300 g spelled flour type 1050
- ½ tsp salt
- 150 g cold butter (diced)
- 1 egg
- 1 ½ tbsp cold water

For the filling:

- 100 g red onions (about 2 medium-sized onions)
- 1 ½ tbsp olive oil
- 100 g chorizo (sliced)
- 160 ml whipped cream
- 120 ml of milk
- 4 eggs
- 80 g Kaltenbach gold (grated, plus more)
- smoked sea salt
- black pepper
- 200 g medium zucchini (1 medium zucchini)
- 80 g ricotta

Preparation steps

1. In a large bowl, put the meal, salt, and cold butter and mix. Then cut the butter with a batter mixer or knife into pieces of pea. Add the egg and a tablespoon of water, mix and knead into a smooth pastry. Add a little more water if the dough does not stick together. Place the dough in a fine film for approximately 30 minutes in the refrigerator.

2. Stick a pan (with removable base) of 24 cm smoothly and reserve. Roll the dough off a bit larger than the shape, then put in the shape and press on both sides. The dough may be too much cut out across the edge. Prick the bucket several times and then place another 30 minutes in the refrigerator.

3. During the batter, peel the onion and cut it into rings. When the batter refreshes. Fry it in a saucepan with some olive oil until it is soft and coloured. Retire and put aside from the pan. Thinly cut the chorizo, briefly fry in one pot on each side. The chorizo is rather gray-drain the fried slices on a piece of cooking paper and put aside. Cut the courgettes in thin slices and set aside. With a peeler.

4. To 200 ° C, prepare the oven. Place a piece of bakery paper in the mold on the dough and weigh it down. Remove paper and weight and bake for another 10-15 minutes until the dough turns a nice color golden brown, blind-bake for about 15 minutes. Take the oven out and allow it to cool a little.

5. Shrink to 180 ° C the oven's temperature. Mix cream, milk, and rubbed cheese with eggs. Season with a good salt and pepper portion of the mixture. Roll the zucchini on a pre-baked base and spread on top the ricotta and chorizo slices into the spaces with a spoon. Put the egg and cheese on it all evenly and bake 50-55 minutes. The filling should be curdled, and the cheese should have a nice brown gold crust (if all is dark, cover with aluminum foil). Take the oven out and let cool for approximately 10-15 minutes, rub some KALTBACH gold, and serve it warm.

Mirabelle Cake

Preparation: 45 min

Ingredients

- 250 g wholemeal spelled flour

- 65 g maple syrup

- salt

- 3 eggs

- 125 g butter

- 700 g red mirabelle plum

- 100 g marzipan paste

- 125 g small oranges (1 small orange)

- 100 g ground almond kernels

- 1 tsp cinnamon powder

Preparation steps

1. To create a smooth dough shortcut, knead wholemeal spelled flour, maple syrup, 1 salt brush, 1 egg, and butter. Wrap in a film and put about 30 minutes in the refrigerator.

2. Wash, cut, and stone the mirabelle plums in half.

3. Separate the rest of the eggs to fill the marzipan. Beat the egg whites until stiff with a pinch of salt. Squeeze the juice and cut the orange in half. Mix egg yolks and orange juice with marzipan. Remove the almonds in the egg yolk mixture, wrap them with the egg whites.

4. Cut the dough, roll out and line with the molds in size. Just pull an edge. Spread the mixer on top and place the plums on the mirabelle on top with interfaces facing up. Sprinkle cinnamon. In a preheated oven, cook for about 30 minutes at 180oC. Remove the pieces and serve.

Banana and Caramel Tart with a Chocolate Base

Preparation: 30 min

Ingredients

- 300 g whole grain oat biscuit

- 2 tbsp desiccated coconut

- 1 tbsp cocoa powder

- 100 g butter

- 300 g medjool dates

- 300 ml water

- 2 tbsp white almond butter

- 2 pinches vanilla powder

- 1 pinch salt

- 2 bananas

- 100 ml whipped cream

Preparation steps

1. Crumble the biscuits in a freezer bag with the rolling pin and mix with the desiccated coconut and cocoa powder. Melt the butter and mix it with the biscuit mixture. Pour into the cake pan and press down firmly on the bottom and edge. Place in the refrigerator for at least 1 hour.

2. In the meantime, core the dates and puree them with the water, the almond butter, the vanilla powder, and a pinch of salt in a blender.

3. Peel the bananas, cut into slices, and line the cake base with them. Spread the caramel cream from the dates on top and smooth out. Whip the cream until stiff, pour into a piping bag, and sprinkle on the cake in small dots. Serve dusted with cocoa if you like.

Chapter Nine. Frozen Desserts and Ice Cream

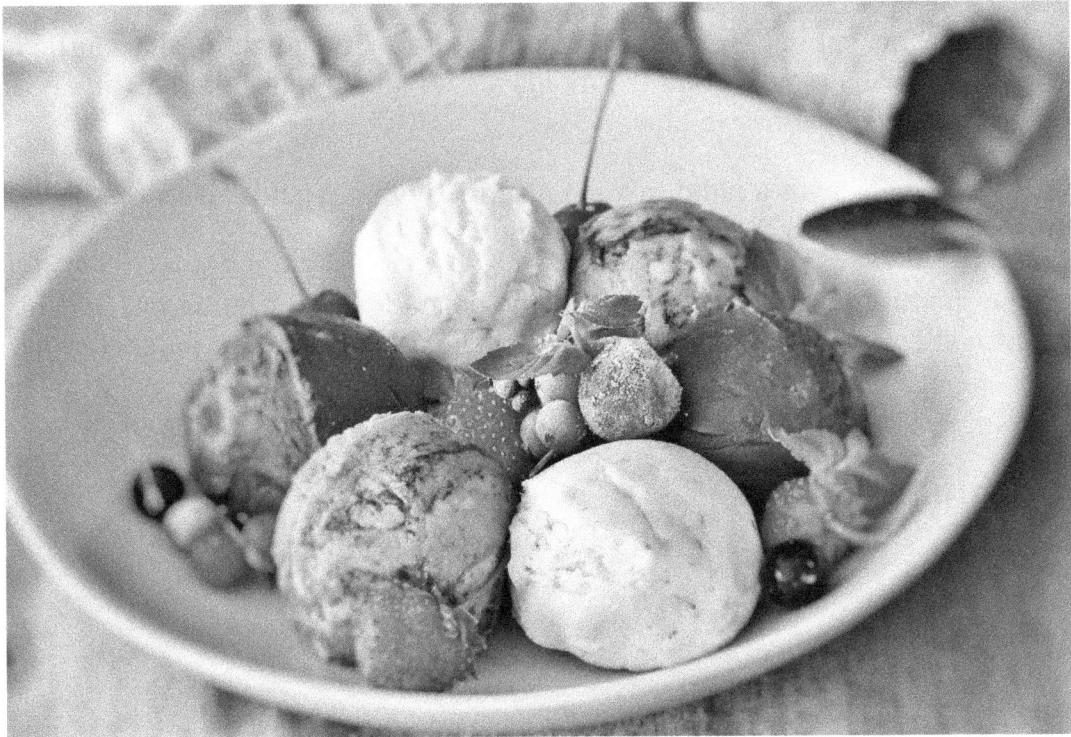

Frozen Blackberry Soufflé

Preparation: 30 min

Ready in 4 h 40 min

Ingredients

- 200 g blackberry
- 2 tbsp honey
- 4 egg yolks
- 125 g cold whipped cream
- soufflé molds
- parchment paper
- adhesive tape

Preparation steps

1. Wash the blackberries and bring them to the boil in a saucepan with honey while stirring. Let simmer for about 5 minutes on low heat. Then let it cool down for 15 minutes.

2. In the meantime, cut out strips of baking paper twice the height of the soufflé molds. Wrap a strip around each mold so that the molds are about 1.5 times the height. Secure the strips of baking paper with adhesive tape.

3. Beat the egg yolks with a hand mixer until lightly foamy and stir in the blackberry puree. Whip the cream until stiff and fold in carefully.

4. Pour the mixture into the molds (up to the edge of the baking paper) and place it in the freezer for at least 4 hours. Remove the strips of parchment paper just before serving.

Frozen Banana Bites

Preparation: 15 minutes

Ready in 1 h 50 min

Ingredients

- 2 bananas

- 1 ½ tbsp peanut butter

- 70 g dark chocolate couverture (at least 70% cocoa content)

Preparation steps

1. Peel the bananas and cut them into finger-thick slices. Brush half of the banana slices with a little peanut butter and cover with the remaining banana pieces. Put in the freezer for about half an hour.

2. Roughly chop the dark chocolate couverture and slowly melt it over a water bath. Take the frozen banana bites out of the freezer. Dip the banana sandwiches halfway into the melted couverture or drizzle with it, place in the freezer again and let freeze for about 1 hour. Let the frozen banana bites thaw for about five minutes before serving.

Chocolate Peanut Ice Cream

Preparation: 15 minutes

Ready in 8 h 15 min

Ingredients

- 4 ripe bananas

- 100 g peanut butter

- 80 ml almond drink (almond milk)

- 40 g dark chocolate (70% cocoa content; vegan)

Preparation steps

1. Peel ripe bananas, cut into slices as thick as a thumb, and freeze for at least 4 hours.

2. Let the bananas thaw briefly, puree with peanut butter and almond drink in a blitz chopper. Alternatively, put in a tall container and puree with a hand blender. Depending on your preference, chop the chocolate coarsely or finely and pour it into the ice cream.

3. Pour nice cream into the moulds and let freeze for about 1 hour. Then insert wooden handles and leave to freeze for another 3 hours. To serve, remove the chocolate-peanut-nice cream from the moulds and enjoy.

Frozen Berry Yoghurt

Ingredients

- 300 g mixed berries e.g. b. strawberries, raspberries, blackberries, and blueberries, as desired

- 2 tbsp lemon juice

- 600 g yoghurt

- 4 tbsp honey

Preparation steps

1. Wash and clean the berries and set some aside for garnish. Finely puree the remaining berries and strain them through a sieve. Stir a third of the puree with the lemon juice into the yoghurt and sweeten with the honey to taste.

2. Fill the yoghurt into (sturdy) glasses (not full), fill with berry puree, and garnish with berries. Place in the freezer for at least 5 hours. Let thaw for about 15 minutes before serving.

Frozen Strawberry Shake

Preparation: 40 min

Ready in 1 h 10 min

Ingredients

- 250 g strawberries

- 100 ml cherry juice

- 2 tsp sugar

- 2 tbsp lime juice

- 8 tbsp crushed ice

- lemon balm leaf for garnish

Preparation steps

1. Sort the strawberries, wash, and pat dry. Put one strawberry aside for the garnish, layout the rest flat, and let freeze in the freezer for about 30 minutes. Then add the cherry juice, sugar, lime juice, and ice to the blender and puree well.

2. To serve, pour into a glass and garnish with a little lemon balm and a strawberry.

Frozen Melon Skewers

Preparation: 20 min

Ready in 3 h 20 min

Ingredients

- ½ sugar melon
- ½ cantaloupe melon
- ¼ watermelon
- 12 wooden skewers
- 50 ml of lemon juice
- 2 tbsp sugar

Preparation steps

1. Core the melons and poke balls out of the melon with a Parisian cookie cutter. Mix lemon juice with sugar and a little water and add the melon balls.

2. Place the melon balls on the wooden skewers in alternating colours and freeze them lying next to each other on a tray for at least 3 hours.

3. Take out of the freezer for about 5 minutes before serving and arrange on plates.

4. A refreshing treat instead of ice cream.

Ice Cream Cake with Frozen Wild Berries

Ingredients

- 1 kg white couverture
- 400 g mixed, frozen berries (strawberries, blackberries, and blueberries)
- ice
- 150 ml of milk
- 100 g sugar

- 4 egg yolks

- 250 ml whipped cream

- 1 vanilla pod

- 1 cinnamon stick

- 1-star anise

- 20 ml orange liqueur

- 100 ml whipped cream, whipped until half firm

- the chocolate figure at will;

Preparation steps

1. Chop the chocolate and melt it over a hot water bath while stirring. Pour into 5 square chocolate moulds (approx. 12x12 cm) and allow to set (save approx. 50 g of chocolate for later). Then remove them from the moulds and decorate the plates with chocolate figures as desired. The best way to do this is to melt some of the retained chocolate, place swabs on the chocolate bars, and stick the desired figures in this way. Then melt the edges of the chocolate bars (preferably in a not too hot saucepan, press briefly on the bottom) and put them together to form a 'box'. If the corners are not tight, close the holes with the rest of the chocolate.

2. For the ice cream, slit open the vanilla pod, bring to the boil with the cinnamon stick and anise star in the milk.

3. Beat egg yolks with sugar and orange liqueur until frothy and slowly pour in hot milk. Then stir creamy over a hot water bath, remove from heat and beat until cold. Remove the aromatics and carefully fold in the whipped cream. Fill into the prepared "chocolate box" and freeze for at least 4 hours. Spread the berries on the cake about 20 minutes before serving and let them thaw. Decorate with a ribbon if you like.

Frozen Lime Margarita

Preparation: 10 min

Ingredients

- 40 ml tequila
- ½ lime juice
- 20 ml rose's lime juice
- 6 tbsp crushed ice
- lime juice
- salt

Preparation steps

1. Put some ice cubes in a blender, add tequila, lime fillets, and lime juice and mix quickly to a creamy consistency.

2. Moisten the rim of a cocktail bowl with lime juice, then dip in salt. Pour frozen margarita into the glass. Garnish with a lime wedge if you like.

Chapter Ten. Custard and Mousse

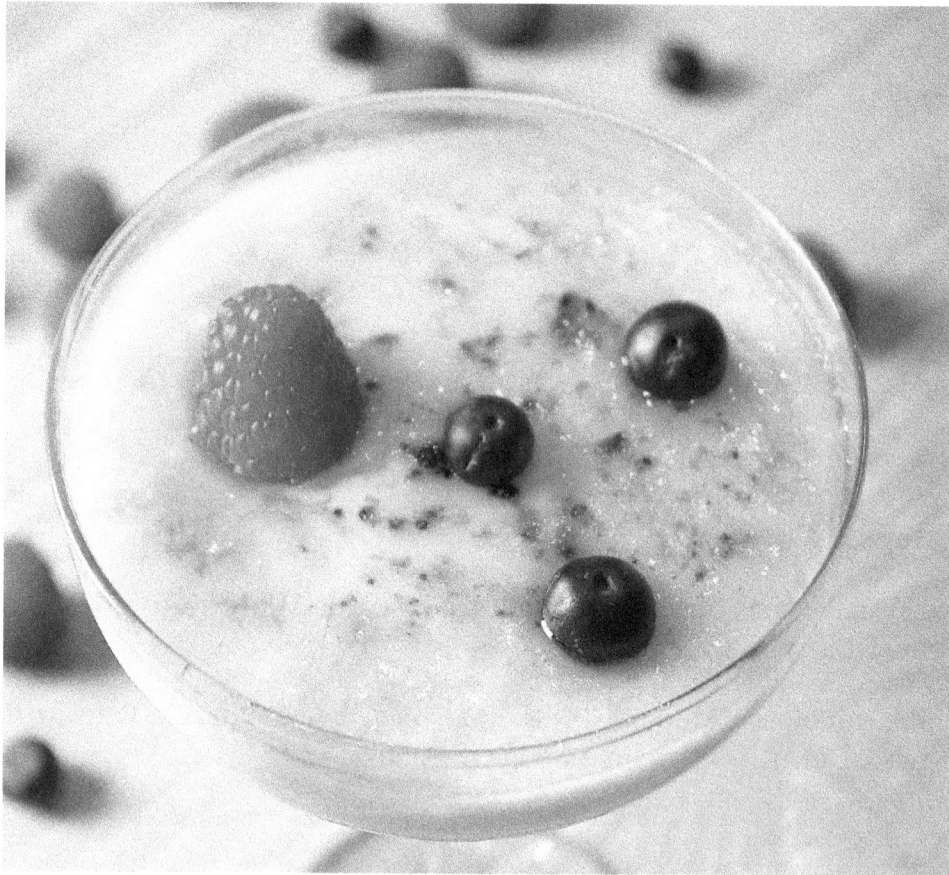

Custard with Cherries

Ingredients

- 800 g cherries

- 50 g ground hazelnuts

- 4 eggs

- 50 g sugar

- 1 tbsp vanilla sugar

- 50 g flour

- 275 ml of milk

- ½ tsp cinnamon powder

- butter for the mould

- icing sugar for dusting

Preparation steps

1. Wash, pat dry, and stone the cherries. Preheat the oven to 180 ° C.

2. Toast the hazelnuts in a pan without fat. Let cool down. Separate the eggs. Beat the egg yolks with the sugar and vanilla sugar until creamy white. Stir in the milk, cinnamon, nuts, and flour (batter should not be too runny). Beat the egg whites until stiff and fold in. Finally, mix in the cherries and put everything in an ovenproof baking pan (approx. 2 liters). Place in a drip pan, pour hot water (about halfway through the baking pan), and carefully place in the oven. Bake until golden brown for about 40 minutes. Serve hot or cold dusted with powdered sugar.

Baked Apple with Custard

Preparation: 30 min

Ingredients

- 4 sour apples

- 75 g rated almond kernels

- 3 tsp raisins

- 45 g maple syrup (3 tbsp)

- 1 pinch ground cinnamon

- 50 g marzipan paste

- 20 g butter in pieces

- 250 ml milk (3.5% fat)

- 1 vanilla pod

- 1 tsp food starch

- 3 egg yolks

Preparation steps

1. Wash the apples and use an apple cutter to poke out the core.

2. For the filling, mix half of the almonds with the raisins, 1 tbsp maple syrup, and cinnamon, finely chop the marzipan mixture, and stir in. Fill the apples with it and put them in a baking dish. Sprinkle with the remaining almonds. Spread pieces of butter on top and bake in a preheated oven at 200 ° C (convection 180 ° C; gas: level 3) for 30–40 minutes.

3. In the meantime, remove 3–4 tablespoons from the milk for the vanilla sauce and stir until smooth with the starch. Halve the vanilla pod lengthways, scrape out the vanilla pulp with a knife and bring the vanilla pod and pulp to the boil in the remaining milk. Take off the stove.

4. Whisk the cornstarch with the egg yolk and the milk you set aside, stir into the vanilla milk, and heat while stirring (do not boil) until the vanilla sauce is creamy. Season to taste with the rest of the maple syrup, allow to cool a little, and stir occasionally.

5. Take the baked apple out of the oven, arrange on plates, and serve with lukewarm vanilla sauce.

Tart with Pudding Filling

Preparation: 40 min

Ingredients

For the dough

- 250 g flour

- 75 g sugar

- 1 pinch salt

- 1 tsp lemon peel

- 1 egg

- 160 g butter

- flour for the work surface

- legumes for sprinkling

For covering

- 5 eggs

- 150 g sugar

- 150 g cream double

- 400 ml of milk

- 1 vanilla pod scraped pulp

- 75 g butter

Preparation steps

1. Mix the flour with sugar, salt, and lemon zest, place on the worktop, place a cavity in the center, beat the egg, and spread the butter in flakes around the cavity. Work quickly with your hands to form a smooth dough, form a ball, wrap in foil and refrigerate for 30 minutes.

2. Preheat the oven to 180 ° C with a higher and lower temperature.

3. Roll out the dough on a floured surface slightly larger than the mold and place it on the pan with butter. Pull one end, prick the base several times with a fork, cover with baking paper and sprinkle with legumes. Bake blindly in a preheated oven for about 15 minutes.

4. Meanwhile, in a metal bowl, beat the eggs and sugar until foam, add cream, milk, and vanilla pulp and add the butter in small flakes, then beat in a double boiler with a hand blender until thick, creamy consistency.

5. Take the base out of the oven, remove the legumes and parchment paper, and let the base cool slightly. Spread the egg cream on top, smooth it, and bake in a preheated oven for about 30-35 minutes. Cover with buttered baking paper so that the surface is not too golden.

6. Remove the baked cake from the oven, cool, carefully remove it from the pan and serve cut into pieces.

Cookies with Chocolate Filling

Preparation: 50 min

Ingredients

- 250 g cream cheese
- 200 g dark chocolate at least 70% cocoa content
- 1 tsp honey
- 100 g spelled flour type 1050
- 100 g wholemeal spelled flour
- 100 g ground almond
- 80 g coconut blossom sugar
- ½ vanilla pod
- 1 egg (size m)
- 200 g butter

Preparation steps

1. For the filling, finely chop the dark chocolate and melt it in a small saucepan with the honey. Take the pot off the stove and let it cool slightly. Mix in the cream cheese with a whisk, then let the cream rest in the refrigerator.

2. Meanwhile, scrape out the pulp of the vanilla, mix the flour with the almonds, coconut blossom sugar, and vanilla pulp and pile them on a countertop. Make a well in the middle, beat in the egg and distribute the butter in flakes around the well. Use your hands to quickly work all the ingredients into a smooth dough, shape into a ball, and wrap in the fridge for about 1 hour.

3. Line the baking sheets with parchment paper. Roll out the dough on a lightly floured work surface approx. 4 mm thin, cut out a circle with a diameter of approx. 3 cm and place it on the baking paper with a gap. Bake in a preheated oven at 180 ° C (convection: 160 ° C; gas: level 2–3) for 8–10 minutes until light. Then take out and let cool on a wire rack.

4. Take the filling out of the refrigerator, beat well with the hand mixer, pour into a piping bag with a star nozzle, and squirt onto half of the cookies. Put the other half together and dust with powdered sugar if you like. Spread the rest of the cream on the cookies as a swab, store in a cool place, and consume quickly.

Chocolate Coconut Cream

Preparation: 20 min

Ingredients

- 400 g yoghurt alternative made from almond kernels
- 40 g coconut blossom sugar
- 100 g coconut cream
- 35 g desiccated coconut
- 55 g cocoa powder
- mint for garnish

Preparation steps

1. Mix the yoghurt alternative with coconut blossom sugar until smooth. Mix half with 75 g coconut cream and desiccated coconut. Mix the second half with the remaining coconut cream and 2 tbsp cocoa until smooth.

2. Wash the mint leaves and shake dry. Pour both materials into a piping bag with a large star nozzle. Divide 1 teaspoon of cocoa powder into four glasses. First, spray the chocolate cream on the cocoa. Then finish with the light cream. Finally, dust with a little cocoa powder and serve

Strawberry Cream

Ingredients

- 300 g strawberries
- 20 ml strawberry liqueur
- 150 g yoghurt
- 150 g whipped cream
- sugar to taste
- 4 sheets gelatin white
- 2 sheets gelatin red

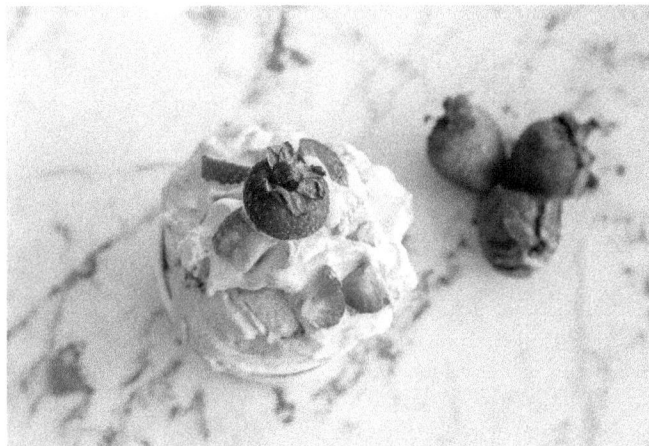

Preparation steps

1. Soak the gelatine in plenty of cold water. Wash, clean, and finely puree the strawberries. Brush through a sieve. Mix the yoghurt with the strawberries and a little sugar to taste until smooth, season to taste. Squeeze out the gelatine, melt it in a small saucepan at a mild temperature and stir in some yoghurt cream. (Temperature compensation)

2. Quickly stir the mixed gelatine into the rest of the cream, add the liqueur, stir in and let it gel. Whip the cream very stiff, as soon as the cream starts to gel, fold in and pour into 4 glasses, chill.

Vegan Chocolate Mousse

Ingredients

- 2 cups simply v spreading pleasure creamy-mild

- 100 ml coconut milk

- 4 tbsp agave syrup

- 2 tbsp cocoa powder

- 100 g dark chocolate

Preparation steps

1. In a bowl, stir the Simply V Streichgenuss Creamy Mild with coconut milk until creamy. Fold in agave syrup, cocoa powder, and melted chocolate until smooth.

2. Fill into glasses and refrigerate for at least 2 hours. To serve, decorate with a yogurt alternative, banana slices, grated chocolate, and nuts, depending on your taste.

Rhubarb Creme

Ingredients

- 500 g strawberry rhubarb
- vanilla pod
- 6 sheets gelatin
- 100 g coconut blossom sugar
- egg white (very fresh)
- 100 ml whipped cream

Preparation steps

1. Clean the rhubarb and cut into small pieces. Cut the vanilla pod lengthways and scrape out the pulp. Soak the gelatine in plenty of cold water. Put the rhubarb pieces in a saucepan with 50 ml water, 50 g coconut blossom sugar, and vanilla pulp and bring to the boil. Simmer over a very low heat for about 10 minutes, then puree finely and reheat. Add gelatine to the mashed rhubarb while dripping wet, dissolve while stirring, and chill the mixture.

2. Beat the egg whites until stiff, drizzling in the remaining coconut blossom sugar. Whip the cream until stiff too. As soon as the rhubarb mixture begins to gel, fold in the cream, then fold in the egg whites, but do not mix too much so that a marble pattern can be seen. Pour the rhubarb cream into 6 dessert bowls and place in the refrigerator until ready to serve.

Red Macarons with Chocolate Cream

Preparation: 35 min

Ingredients

For the macarons

- 100 g raspberries
- 270 g powdered sugar
- 4 protein
- 2 tsp lemon juice

- 200 g peeled ground almond kernels

- red food coloring at will

For the filling

- 220 g dark chocolate couverture

- 120 ml whipped cream

- 40 g butter

Preparation steps

1. For the macarons, rinse, pat dry and puree the raspberries. Strain the raspberry puree through a fine sieve and mix well with 2 tablespoons of powdered sugar.

2. Beat the egg whites with the lemon juice until stiff, gradually fold in the icing sugar until you have a stiff, shiny mixture. Carefully fold the almonds and raspberry puree into the egg whites. Add some food coloring for an intense red color.

3. Preheat the oven to 150 ° C and line a baking sheet with parchment paper. Fill a piping bag with a large, round opening with the cream. Squirt small hemispheres about 2 cm in diameter onto the tray. Bake in the oven for about 25 minutes, leave the oven ajar (e.g. stick a wooden spoon in the oven door). Remove the macarons and let them cool down.

4. For the chocolate filling, chop the couverture into small pieces and carefully melt in a water bath. Whip the cream until creamy. Mix the butter in small pieces with the whisk into the melted chocolate. As soon as the chocolate has cooled, fold in the cream. Pour into a piping bag and sprinkle half of the macarons with the filling on the flat bottom. Then combine with the remaining macarons.

Chapter Eleven. Shakes and Smoothies

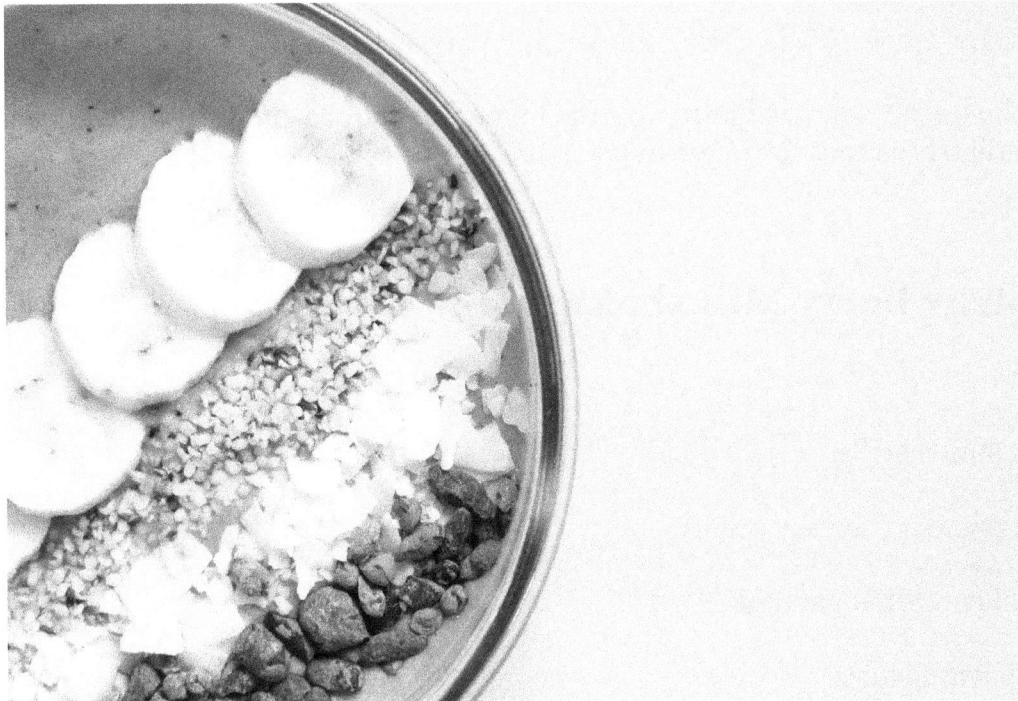

Healthy Green Shot

Preparation: 15 minutes

Ingredients

- 2 pears

- 3 green apples (e.g. granny smith)

- 3 poles celery

- 60 g organic ginger

- parsley (20 g)

- kiwi fruit

- limes

- 1 tsp turmeric

Preparation steps

1. Wash pears, apples, celery, ginger, and parsley and cut into pieces. Halve the kiwi fruit and remove the pulp with a spoon. Halve the limes and squeeze out the juice.

2. Put pears, apples, kiwis, celery, ginger, and parsley in the juicer and squeeze out the juice.

3. Mix the freshly squeezed juice with the lime juice and season with turmeric. Serve mixture immediately as shots or freeze in portions.

Vegan Strawberry Milkshake

Ingredients

- 250 g strawberries

- 150 g unsweetened soy yogurt

- 150 ml oat drink (oat milk)

- splash lemon juice

- 1 pinch vanilla powder

Preparation steps

1. Wash, clean and halve the strawberries; Put 2 strawberry halves aside.

2. Finely puree the remaining strawberries with soy yoghurt, oat drink, lemon juice, and vanilla powder in a blender.

3. Divide the vegan strawberry milkshake between 2 glasses and garnish with the strawberry halves that were set aside.

Kiwi Milkshake

Ingredients

- 3 kiwi fruit
- tbsp honey
- tbsp lemon juice
- 300 ml milk (3.5% fat)
- crushed ice

Preparation steps

1. Peel and roughly chop the kiwifruit and puree with honey and lemon juice. Pour in some milk and puree the drink again.

2. Pour crushed ice and kiwi milkshake into 2 tall glasses and serve.

Kale and Ginger Smoothie

Ingredients

- 200 g pineapple pulp
- ½ lemon
- 100 g tender kale leaf
- box cress
- 10 g ginger (1 piece)
- 300 ml coconut water

Preparation steps

1. Cut the pineapple into pieces. Squeeze the lemon half.

2. Clean, wash, and cut the kale. Cut the cress from the bed, set aside for garnish. Peel the ginger and cut into small pieces.

3. Put the pineapple, lemon juice, kale, cress, and ginger in a blender. Pour in coconut water and 200–300 ml of water and puree.

4. Fill the smoothie into glasses and serve with the remaining cress.

Grape Shake

Ingredients

- 150 g red grapes
- tsp lemon juice
- 1 tbsp honey
- 1 tbsp yeast flakes
- 300 ml chilled buttermilk
- mint to garnish

Preparation steps

1. Rinse the grapes, clean them, cut them in half and core if you like, put some aside for garnish. Put lemon juice, honey, and yeast flakes in the blender or puree with the cutting stick of the hand mixer

2. Gradually mix in the buttermilk. Pour into two tall glasses and decorate with fresh grapes and mint leaves.

Smoothie with Melon

Ingredients

- 250 g watermelon pulp
- 150 g cherry tomatoes
- 2 handfuls basil
- salt
- pepper from the mill

Preparation steps

1. Roughly dice the melon pulp. Wash and halve the tomatoes. Wash the basil and shake dry. Put everything together with 100 ml of water in the mixer and puree finely.

2. Depending on the desired consistency, add a little more water. Season to taste with salt and pepper, fill into glasses and serve garnished with basil.

Fruity Herbal Smoothie

Ingredients

- 150 g spinach

- 2 handfuls mixed herbs (e.g. chervil, mint, tarragon, parsley)

- 2 apples

- orange

- 1 tsp olive oil

- 500 ml of mineral water

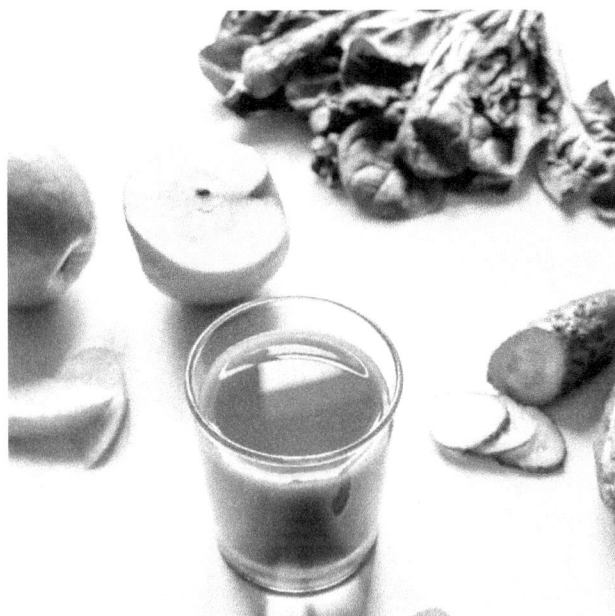

Preparation steps

1. Clean and wash the spinach and herbs and spin dry. Put some herbs aside. Wash, peel, core and cut the apples into large pieces. Squeeze the orange.

2. Puree the spinach, herbs, apple pieces and orange juice in a blender. Add oil and fill up with water. Mix again until foamy and pour the drink into 4 glasses. Serve immediately with straws and the remaining herbs as a garnish.

Carrot Drink

Ingredients

- 2 small cloves of garlic
- 800 g bunch of carrots
- flat-leaf parsley
- ½ lemon
- 1 tsp rapeseed oil

Preparation steps

1. Peel the garlic cloves.
2. Wash the carrots thoroughly and cut off the ends.
3. Wash the parsley and shake dry. Squeeze the lemon half.
4. Juice the garlic and 6 carrots in the juicer.
5. Put the parsley and remaining carrots in the juicer and extract the juice.
6. Mix the carrot drink with about 2 tablespoons of lemon juice and the rapeseed oil and enjoy immediately.

Blackberry and Peach Cocktail

Ingredients

- 200 g large ripe peaches (1 large ripe peach)
- 200 g blackberry (frozen or fresh)
- 100 ml mineral water (ice cold)

Preparation steps

1. Wash the peach, pat dry, cut in half and remove the stone. Quarter peach; Cut 2-3 thin slices from a quarter and set aside. If necessary, sort fresh berries, rinse and pat dry.
2. Dice the rest of the peach and finely puree with the berries in a blender. (Add frozen fruit, not defrosted.)

3. Put the puree in a glass and fill up with mineral water. Garnish with the peach slices.

Banana Shake

Ingredients

- 2 bananas
- 400 ml oat drink (oat milk)
- vanilla pod

Preparation steps

1. Peel the bananas and put them in a blender with the oat drink. Cut the vanilla pod lengthways, scrape out the pulp and add.

2. Mix well and pour into two tall glasses. For example, serve as a snack with some banana slices.

Avocado Yoghurt Drink

Ingredients

- large ripe avocado
- 20 g basil (1 bunch)
- tsp lemon juice
- 400 g yoghurt (3.5% fat)
- 100 ml milk (3.5% fat)
- salt
- pepper

Preparation steps

1. Peel, halve, core and cut the avocado into pieces.

2. Wash the basil, shake dry and pluck the leaves.

3. Roughly chop half of the leaves.

4. Finely puree the avocado with lemon juice, chopped basil leaves, yoghurt and milk in a blender. Season to taste with salt and pepper. Fill into 4 glasses and garnish with the remaining basil leaves.

Mango Smoothie Bowl with Kiwi

Ingredients

- mango

- ½ yellow pepper

- 1 lemon

- 100 ml orange juice

- kiwi fruit

- 10 g pistachio nuts (2 teaspoons)

- 10 g flaxseed (2 tsp)

- 30 g cranberries (2 tbsp; sweetened with juice)

Preparation steps

1. Peel the mango, remove the pulp from the stone and cut into small pieces. Clean, wash and chop the peppers. Halve the lemon and squeeze out the juice. Put the mango, paprika, orange and lemon juice in a blender and puree finely. Divide the smoothie into 4 bowls.

2. For the topping, peel, halve and slice the kiwi fruit. Chop the pistachios. Place the kiwi slices, pistachios, linseeds and cranberries decoratively on the smoothie bowls.

Peach Yoghurt Drink

Ingredients

- 125 g ripe peaches (1 ripe peach)

- 50 g yoghurt (0.3% fat)

- 50 ml coconut milk (1.9% fat; health food store)

- 100 ml of mineral water (ice cold)

- pinch saffron threads

Preparation steps

1. Rinse the peach, dip briefly in boiling water, rinse with cold water and peel off the skin. Then halve, stone and dice.

2. Put the peach cubes with yoghurt and coconut milk in a tall container and puree finely with a hand blender.

3. Pour into a glass and add the mineral water. Add ice cubes and sprinkle with saffron.

Pear and Lime Marmalade

Ingredients for 1.5 l jam:

- 3-4 untreated limes

- 1 kg ripe pears

- 500 g jam sugar 2: 1

Preparation Steps

1. Wash 2 limes and grate dry.

2. Peel the peels thinly with the zest ripper.

3. Then cut all limes in half and squeeze them out. Measure out 100 ml of lime juice. Wash and peel the pears, remove the core and then quarter them. Weigh 900 g of pulp. Then puree the pears together with the lime juice.

4. Now put the pear puree together with the lime peels and the jellied sugar in a saucepan. Bring all ingredients to the boil together.

5. Simmer for 4 minutes, stirring, taking care not to burn anything. Make a gelation test with a small blob on a cold saucer. If this becomes solid in a short time, the jam is ready. Remove any foam that may have formed with a trowel, but you can also simply stir it in.

6. Then pour the hot mass into hot rinsed jars, close and let stand upside down.

Peach Yogurt Drink with Coconut Milk

Ingredients

- 125 g ripe peaches (1 ripe peach)

- 50 g yogurt (0.3% fat)

- 50 ml coconut milk (1.9% fat; health food store)

- 100 ml mineral water (ice cold)

- 1 pinch

- saffron threads

Preparation steps

1. Rinse the peach, dip briefly in boiling water, rinse with cold water and peel off the skin.

2. Then halve, stone and dice. Put the peach cubes with yoghurt and coconut milk in a tall container and puree finely with a hand blender. Pour into a glass and add the mineral water.

3. Add ice cubes and sprinkle with saffron.

Lightning Source UK Ltd.
Milton Keynes UK
UKHW050736080121
376670UK00013B/1435